Advances in Maternal Fetal Medicine

Editors

CYNTHIA GYAMFI-BANNERMAN
RUSSELL MILLER

CLINICS IN PERINATOLOGY

www.perinatology.theclinics.com

Consulting Editor
LUCKY JAIN

December 2020 • Volume 47 • Number 4

ELSEVIER

1600 John F. Kennedy Boulevard • Suite 1800 • Philadelphia, Pennsylvania, 19103-2899

http://www.theclinics.com

CLINICS IN PERINATOLOGY Volume 47, Number 4
December 2020 ISSN 0095-5108, ISBN-13: 978-0-323-76481-0

Editor: Kerry Holland
Developmental Editor: Casey Potter

Clinics in Perinatology (ISSN 0095-5108) is published quarterly by Elsevier Inc., 360 Park Avenue South, New York, NY 10010-1710. Months of issue are March, June, September, and December. Business and Editorial Offices: 1600 John F. Kennedy Blvd., Ste. 1800, Philadelphia, PA 19103-2899. Customer Service Office: 3251 Riverport Lane, Maryland Heights, MO 63043. Periodicals postage paid at New York, NY and additional mailing offices. Subscription prices are $312.00 per year (US individuals), $610.00 per year (US institutions), $365.00 per year (Canadian individuals), $747.00 per year (Canadian institutions), $435.00 per year (international individuals), $747.00 per year (international institutions), $100.00 per year (US and Canadian students), and $195.00 per year (International students). International air speed delivery is included in all Clinics subscription prices. All prices are subject to change without notice. **POSTMASTER:** Send address changes to *Clinics in Perinatology*, Elsevier Health Sciences Division, Subscription Customer Service, 3251 Riverport Lane, Maryland Heights, MO 63043. **Customer Service: Telephone: 1-800-654-2452** (U.S. and Canada); **1-314-447-8871** (outside U.S. and Canada). **Fax: 1-314-447-8029. E-mail: journalscustomerservice-usa@elsevier.com** (for print support); **journalsonlinesupport-usa@elsevier.com** (for online support).

Reprints. For copies of 100 or more, of articles in this publication, please contact the Commercial Reprints Department, Elsevier Inc., 360 Park Avenue South, New York, NY 10010-1710. Tel. 212-633-3874; Fax: 212-633-3820; E-mail: reprints@elsevier.com.

Clinics in Perinatology is also published in Spanish by McGraw-Hill Interamericana Editores S.A., P.O. Box 5-237, 06500 Mexico D.F., Mexico.

Clinics in Perinatology is covered in *MEDLINE/PubMed (Index Medicus) Current Contents, Excepta Medica, BIOSIS and ISI/BIOMED.*

Printed in the United States of America.

Contributors

CONSULTING EDITOR

LUCKY JAIN, MD
George W. Brumley Jr Professor and Chair, Emory University School of Medicine, Department of Pediatrics, Chief Academic Officer, Children's Healthcare of Atlanta, Executive Director, Emory+Children's Pediatric Institute, Atlanta, Georgia, USA

EDITORS

CYNTHIA GYAMFI-BANNERMAN, MD, MSc
Vice Chair for Faculty Development, Ellen Jacobson Levine and Eugene Jacobson Professor of OBGYN, Director, Maternal Fetal Medicine Fellowship Program, Co-Director, CUIMC Preterm Birth Prevention Center, Department of Obstetrics and Gynecology, Columbia University Irving Medical Center, New York, New York

RUSSELL MILLER, MD
Sloane Hospital for Women Associate Professor of Prenatal Pediatrics (in Obstetrics and Gynecology), Medical Director, Carmen and John Thain Center for Prenatal Pediatrics, Division of Maternal Fetal Medicine, Department of Obstetrics and Gynecology, Columbia University Irving Medical Center, New York, New York

AUTHORS

WHITNEY A. BOOKER, MD, MS
Division of Maternal Fetal Medicine, Department of Obstetrics and Gynecology, College of Physicians and Surgeons, Columbia University Irving Medical Center, New York, New York

ANN E.B. BORDERS, MD, MSc, MPH
Clinical Associate Professor, Feinberg School of Medicine, Center for Healthcare Services and Outcomes Research, Institute for Population Health and Medicine, Northwestern University, Pritzker School of Medicine, University of Chicago, Chicago, Illinois; Division of Maternal Fetal Medicine, Department of Obstetrics and Gynecology, NorthShore University HealthSystem, Evanston, Illinois

NOELLE BRESLIN, MD
Fellow, Division of Maternal Fetal Medicine, Columbia University Irving Medical Center, New York Presbyterian Hospital, New York, New York

UKACHI N. EMERUWA, MD, MPH
Division of Maternal Fetal Medicine, Department of Obstetrics and Gynecology, Columbia University Irving Medical Center, New York, New York

ALEXANDER FRIEDMAN, MD
Associate Professor of Obstetrics and Gynecology, Division of Maternal Fetal Medicine, Department of Obstetrics and Gynecology, College of Physicians and Surgeons, Columbia University, New York, New York

CYNTHIA GYAMFI-BANNERMAN, MD, MSc
Vice Chair for Faculty Development, Ellen Jacobson Levine and Eugene Jacobson Professor of OBGYN, Director, Maternal Fetal Medicine Fellowship Program, Co-Director, CUIMC Preterm Birth Prevention Center, Department of Obstetrics and Gynecology, Columbia University Irving Medical Center, New York, New York

IBRAHIM HAMMAD, MD, MSCI
Assistant Professor, Maternal Fetal Medicine, Intermountain Healthcare and the University of Utah, Salt Lake City, Utah

ZSAKEBA T. HENDERSON, MD
Medical Officer, Division of Reproductive Health, National Center for Chronic Disease Prevention and Health Promotion, Centers for Disease Control and Prevention, Atlanta, Georgia

BRENNA L. HUGHES, MD, MSc
Duke University Hospital, Durham, North Carolina

ADINA R. KERN-GOLDBERGER, MD, MPH
Department of Obstetrics and Gynecology, Maternal Child Health Research Center, University of Pennsylvania Perelman School of Medicine, Hospital of the University of Pennsylvania, Philadelphia, Pennsylvania

NICOLE M. KRENITSKY, MD, MBA
Department of Obstetrics and Gynecology, Columbia University Irving Medical Center, New York, New York

RUTH LANDAU, MD
Professor, Department of Anesthesiology, Columbia University Irving Medical Center, New York, New York

PATRICIA ANN LEE KING, PhD, MSW
Senior Research Associate, Feinberg School of Medicine, Center for Healthcare Studies and Outcomes Research, Institute for Public Health and Medicine, Northwestern University, Pritzker School of Medicine, University of Chicago, Chicago, Illinois

RUSSELL MILLER, MD
Sloane Hospital for Women Associate Professor of Prenatal Pediatrics (in Obstetrics and Gynecology), Medical Director, Carmen and John Thain Center for Prenatal Pediatrics, Division of Maternal Fetal Medicine, Department of Obstetrics and Gynecology, Columbia University Irving Medical Center, New York, New York

T. FLINT PORTER, MD
Maternal Fetal Medicine, Intermountain Healthcare and the University of Utah, Salt Lake City, Utah

LAUREN SAYRES, MD
University of Colorado, Aurora, Colorado

BEN SHATIL, DO, MPH
Assistant Professor, Department of Anesthesiology, Emory University Hospital Midtown, Atlanta, Georgia

JEAN-JU SHEEN, MD
Division of Maternal Fetal Medicine, Department of Obstetrics and Gynecology, Columbia University Irving Medical Center, New York, New York

SINDHU K. SRINIVAS, MD, MSCE
Department of Obstetrics and Gynecology, Maternal Child Health Research Center, University of Pennsylvania Perelman School of Medicine, Hospital of the University of Pennsylvania, Philadelphia, Pennsylvania

DESMOND SUTTON, MD
Division of Maternal Fetal Medicine, Department of Obstetrics and Gynecology, College of Physicians and Surgeons, Columbia University, New York, New York

AMY L. TURITZ, MD
Assistant Professor of Obstetrics and Gynecology, Division of Maternal Fetal Medicine, Department of Obstetrics and Gynecology, Columbia University Irving Medical Center, New York, New York

TIMOTHY WEN, MD, MPH
Maternal Fetal Medicine Fellow, Division of Maternal Fetal Medicine, Department of Obstetrics, Gynecology and Reproductive Sciences, University of California, San Francisco, San Francisco, California

Contents

Preterm birth accounts for only 11% of live births but contributes to up to 75% of neonatal mortality and more than half of long-term morbidity. Targeted interventions to reduce the most common causes of perinatal morbidity and mortality include intrapartum group B Streptococcus prophylaxis, magnesium sulfate for fetal neuroprotection, antenatal corticosteroids for fetal lung maturity, latency antibiotics for preterm premature rupture of membranes, and tocolysis to allow corticosteroid administration and transfer to a tertiary care center. This article reviews the evidence for interventions to improve outcomes for fetuses at risk for preterm delivery at different gestational ages.

Preterm birth remains a major issue in obstetrics. Despite efforts to reduce the incidence of preterm delivery, rates in the United States remain high at 10.2% of all live births with an incidence of 10.8% globally. Preterm birth is the leading cause of neonatal morbidity and mortality worldwide. It is also the leading cause of death in children younger than 5 years. Research into this important health topic has allowed for the identification of risk factors for preterm birth, the most important of which is a history of prior preterm birth. Cervical length screening may allow us to identify those at greatest risk of recurrent preterm birth as well as a de novo risk in women with no prior preterm birth history.

Monochorionic twin gestations possess disproportionately higher risk for perinatal morbidity and mortality when compared with dichorionic twin pregnancies due to their potential to develop specific complications attributable to a shared placenta and intertwin placental circulation. Since the advent of fetoscopic laser surgery, outcomes of pregnancies affected by twin-twin transfusion syndrome (TTTS) have improved, with reduced rates of mortality and morbidity when compared with amnioreduction or expectant management. The focus of this article is to review the literature

withdrawal syndrome, intrauterine growth restriction, neural tube defects, stillbirth, increased maternal mortality, greater postpartum pain, and longer inpatient stays. Patient education about the risks and benefits of multimodal analgesia and empowering shared decision making may help curb the opioid epidemic. Tailoring pain management to individual needs might be the solution to the problem.

Lauren Sayres and Brenna L. Hughes

Understanding the pathophysiology, management, and prevention of emerging infectious diseases among pregnant women is imperative to achieve a successful response from the medical community. Ebola and Zika viruses represent infections with profound public health implications. In particular, Ebola virus is associated with high case fatality and pregnancy and neonatal loss rates, while Zika virus has been associated with multiple congenital anomalies; these features present critical clinical dilemmas for management of pregnant and reproductive aged women. The objective of this article is to summarize key background information and best practices for management of Ebola and Zika virus in pregnancy.

PROGRAM OBJECTIVE

The goal of *Clinics in Perinatology* is to keep practicing perinatologists, neonatologists, obstetricians, practicing physicians and residents up to date with current clinical practice in perinatology by providing timely articles reviewing the state of the art in patient care.

TARGET AUDIENCE

Perinatologists, neonatologists, obstetricians, practicing physicians, residents and healthcare professionals who provide patient care utilizing findings from *Clinics in Perinatology*.

LEARNING OBJECTIVES

Upon completion of this activity, participants will be able to:

1. Review the current evidence, strategies and interventions used to improve outcomes for fetuses at risk for preterm delivery, pediatric survivors of twin-twin transfusion syndrome, and those pregnancies affected by Ebola and Zika virus as well as the use of opioids and immunosuppressive agents in pregnancy.
2. Discuss the role telecommunication tools, shared decision making, and multi-disciplinary team approaches play in improving maternal and neonatal care and outcomes.
3. Recognize how information collected from commonly used administrative data can be leveraged to improve maternal care and reduce disparities.

ACCREDITATION

The Elsevier Office of Continuing Medical Education (EOCME) is accredited by the Accreditation Council for Continuing Medical Education (ACCME) to provide continuing medical education for physicians.

The EOCME designates this journal-based CME activity for a maximum of 11 *AMA PRA Category 1 Credit*(s)™. Physicians should claim only the credit commensurate with the extent of their participation in the activity.

All other health care professionals requesting continuing education credit for this enduring material will be issued a certificate of participation.

DISCLOSURE OF CONFLICTS OF INTEREST

The EOCME assesses conflict of interest with its instructors, faculty, planners, and other individuals who are in a position to control the content of CME activities. All relevant conflicts of interest that are identified are thoroughly vetted by EOCME for fair balance, scientific objectivity, and patient care recommendations. EOCME is committed to providing its learners with CME activities that promote improvements or quality in healthcare and not a specific proprietary business or a commercial interest.

The planning committee, staff, authors and editors listed below have identified no financial relationships or relationships to products or devices they or their spouse/life partner have with commercial interest related to the content of this CME activity:

Whitney A. Booker, MD, MS; Ann E.B. Borders, MD, MSc, MPH; Noelle Breslin, MD; Regina Chavous-Gibson MSN, RN; Ukachi N. Emeruwa, MD, MPH; Alexander Friedman, MD; Cynthia Gyamfi-Bannerman, MD, MSc; Ibrahim Hammad, MD, MSCI; Zsakeba T. Henderson, MD; Kerry Holland; Lucky Jain; Adina R. Kern-Goldberger, MD, MPH; Patricia Ann Lee King, PhD, MSW; Nicole M. Krenitsky, MD, MBA; Ruth Landau, MD; Russell Miller, MD; Swaminathan Nagarajan; T. Flint Porter, MD; Lauren Sayres, MD; Ben Shatil, DO, MPH; Jean-Ju Sheen, MD; Sindhu K. Srinivas, MD, MSCE; Desmond Sutton, MD; Amy L. Turitz, MD; Timothy Wen, MD, MPH.

The planning committee, staff, authors and editors listed below have identified financial relationships or relationships to products or devices they or their spouse/life partner have with commercial interest related to the content of this CME activity:

Brenna L. Hughes, MD, MSc: consultant/advisor for Merck Sharp & Dohme Corp., a subsidiary of Merck & Co., Inc.

UNAPPROVED/OFF-LABEL USE DISCLOSURE

The EOCME requires CME faculty to disclose to the participants:

1. When products or procedures being discussed are off-label, unlabelled, experimental, and/or investigational (not US Food and Drug Administration [FDA] approved); and
2. Any limitations on the information presented, such as data that are preliminary or that represent ongoing research, interim analyses, and/or unsupported opinions. Faculty may discuss information about

pharmaceutical agents that is outside of FDA-approved labelling. This information is intended solely for CME and is not intended to promote off-label use of these medications. If you have any questions, contact the medical affairs department of the manufacturer for the most recent prescribing information.

TO ENROLL

To enroll in the *Clinics in Perinatology* Continuing Medical Education program, call customer service at 1-800-654-2452 or sign up online at http://www.theclinics.com/home/cme. The CME program is available to subscribers for an additional annual fee of USD 245.00.

METHOD OF PARTICIPATION

In order to claim credit, participants must complete the following:
1. Complete enrolment as indicated above.
2. Read the activity.
3. Complete the CME Test and Evaluation. Participants must achieve a score of 70% on the test. All CME Tests and Evaluations must be completed online.

CME INQUIRIES/SPECIAL NEEDS

For all CME inquiries or special needs, please contact elsevierCME@elsevier.com.

CLINICS IN PERINATOLOGY

SERIES OF RELATED INTEREST

Obstetrics and Gynecology Clinics of North America
https://www.obgyn.theclinics.com/

THE CLINICS ARE AVAILABLE ONLINE!
Access your subscription at:
www.theclinics.com

Foreword

Racial Disparities in Perinatal Outcomes Are a Blight on Our Progress

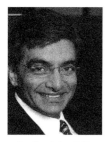

Lucky Jain, MD
Consulting Editor

The year 2020 will remain etched in our memories like none other in recent times. Multiple disruptions have created unprecedented challenges, which have engulfed the entire globe. First, it was the SARS-CoV-2 virus, and the pandemic it caused, that paralyzed every nation, big and small, and brought life as we know it to a standstill. Then came the economic downturn, lost jobs, and businesses turned upside down and their many downstream consequences. And then, particularly for those of us in the United States, unrest related to racial injustice spread like a wildfire. It highlighted the disproportionately high toll COVID-19 has taken on minorities as well as the health disparities that are so pervasive in our environment.

Indeed, births to non-Hispanic black women are associated with a significantly higher risk of prematurity and other adverse outcomes when compared with non-Hispanic white women.[1] A systematic review and metaanalysis by and colleagues[2] showed that black women had a twofold higher risk of preterm birth compared with whites. Similar data can be seen in annual vital statistics year after year and across all preterm gestations (**Fig. 1**).[1] A better understanding of these differences could help shape interventions, but little progress has been made in this regard. Decades ago, David and colleagues[3] showed that black women born in the United States were at greater risk for delivering low-birth-weight babies than women with similar ancestry who had immigrated to the United States from Africa. Studies such as these questioned previously held beliefs about racial differences in birth outcomes resulting from genetic differences and laid bare the consequences of life in the United States as a person of color.[3]

The interplay of social and environmental factors contributing to poorer perinatal outcomes in black women has been the subject of much investigation. Glimmers

Clin Perinatol 47 (2020) xv–xvii
https://doi.org/10.1016/j.clp.2020.09.003
0095-5108/20/© 2020 Published by Elsevier Inc.

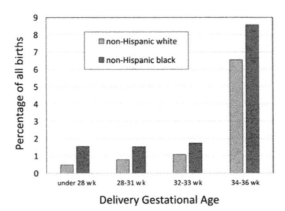

Fig. 1. Proportion of preterm births stratified by gestational age at delivery and maternal race, 2015. *Data from* Martin et al. Final birth data 2015. *From* Manuck TA. Racial and ethnic differences in preterm birth: A complex, multifactorial problem. Semin Perinatol 2017:41;511–518. (Page 517); with permission.

of hope come from "pockets of progress" in certain counties where racial differences in outcomes have all but disappeared (**Fig. 2**).[4] Positive experiences from these areas could and should set the stage for larger public health interventions to remove health disparities once and for all. That will require political will and a societal call for action.

Needless to say, there is more to improving perinatal outcomes than just eliminating racial and health disparities. In this issue of the *Clinics in Perinatology*, Drs Gyamfi-Bannerman and Miller have brought together experts in perinatology to cover topics of great importance in neonatal-perinatal medicine. The authors cover a wide array of topics, including prematurity, infections, maternal conditions, and racial disparities, to name just a few. As always, I am grateful to the publishing staff at Elsevier, including

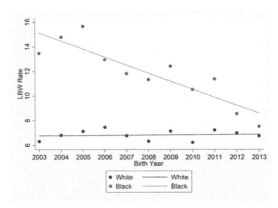

Fig. 2. Aggregated low-birth-weight rates for US counties with convergent racial disparity trend pattern (reductions in black LBW and no increase in white LBW) from 2003-20013. *From* Goldfarb SS, Houser K, Wells BA, Speights JSB, Beitsch L, Rust G. Pockets of progress amidst persistent racial disparities in low birthweight rates. PLoS One 2018: 13(7):e0201658. (page 6/13).

Kerry Holland, Casey Potter, and Nicholas Henderson, for their support in bringing this important publication to you.

Lucky Jain, MD
Department of Pediatrics
Emory University School of Medicine
Children's Healthcare of Atlanta
Emory + Children's Pediatric Institute
2015 Uppergate Drive NE
Atlanta, GA 30322, USA

E-mail address:
ljain@emory.edu

REFERENCES

1. Manuck TA. Racial and ethnic differences in preterm birth: a complex, multifactorial problem. Semin Perinatol 2017;41:511–8.
2. Schaaf JM, Liem SM, Mol BW, et al. Ethnic and racial disparities in the risk of preterm birth: a systematic review and meta-analysis. Am J Perinatol 2013;30:433–50.
3. David RJ, Collins JW Jr. Differing birth weight among infants of US born blacks, African-born blacks, and US-born whites. N Engl J Med 1997;337:1209–14.
4. Goldfarb SS, Houser K, Wells BA, et al. Pockets of progress amidst persistent racial disparities in low birthweight rates. PLoS One 2018;13(7):e0201658.

Preface

Updates in Maternal Fetal Medicine

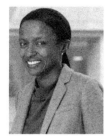 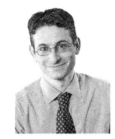

Cynthia Gyamfi-Bannerman, MD, MSc   Russell Miller, MD
Editors

The practice of medicine is continuously evolving, but the changes we experienced while preparing this issue of *Clinics in Perinatology*, during the COVID-19 pandemic, were beyond what we ever expected. The articles were planned prior to the pandemic but completed during the peak of it. With deepest gratitude, we want to thank the generous authors for making this a truly spectacular issue. We cover the breadth and depth of maternal and fetal medicine and hope to include something for everyone. The issue begins with an article on management of preterm pregnancies at risk for delivery, including the use of magnesium and antibiotics. This is followed by an article on preterm birth prevention strategies for women identified to be at risk. We move from preterm birth to complicated monochorionic, diamniotic twin pregnancies and discuss neurologic outcomes after prenatal treatment of twin-twin transfusion syndrome. Moving to the mother in the maternal fetal dyad, we provide an update on the use of biologic agents in pregnancy. Telemedicine became used broadly during the pandemic, and we cover that here, with a comprehensive article on telehealth and obstetrics. Our issue would be incomplete if we did not address racial and socioeconomic disparities in obstetrics, penned by an author who has done much work in this area. We leverage the expertise of our obstetric anesthesia colleagues for the article on opioid use and misuse in pregnancy. We switch gears to statewide and national quality initiatives, describing how this work has led to improved obstetric outcomes around the country. We provide updated guidelines on delivery timing and mode of delivery at term, a topic that is ever the controversy. Or next foray is into hypertensive disorders of pregnancy, understanding newer definitions and evidence-based management strategies. Finally, we discuss rarer infectious diseases during pregnancy, namely Ebola and Zika. We hope that there is something for everyone in this issue, whether your

Clin Perinatol 47 (2020) xix–xx
https://doi.org/10.1016/j.clp.2020.09.002   **perinatology.theclinics.com**
0095-5108/20/© 2020 Published by Elsevier Inc.

background is in obstetrics, in maternal fetal medicine, in neonatology, or from an un-related field. Thanks for reading!

Cynthia Gyamfi-Bannerman, MD, MSc
Department of Obstetrics & Gynecology
Columbia University Irving Medical Center
622 West 168th Street, PH 16-66
New York, NY 10032, USA

Russell Miller, MD
Division of Maternal Fetal Medicine
Department of Obstetrics & Gynecology
Columbia University Irving Medical Center
622 West 168th Street, PH 16-66
New York, NY 10032, USA

E-mail addresses:
cg2231@cumc.columbia.edu (C. Gyamfi-Bannerman)
rsm20@cumc.columbia.edu (R. Miller)

Advances in Management for Preterm Fetuses at Risk of Delivery

Ukachi N. Emeruwa, MD, MPH[a], Nicole M. Krenitsky, MD, MBA[b],
Jean-Ju Sheen, MD[a],*

KEYWORDS

- Preterm birth • Periviability • Betamethasone • Tocolysis • Neuroprotection
- Latency antibiotics • GBS

KEY POINTS

- Increasing rates of preterm birth and very early preterm infant survival contribute disproportionately to short-term and long-term newborn complications.
- Interventions targeted at reducing perinatal morbidity and mortality associated with preterm birth have advanced significantly.
- High-quality evidence supports intrapartum prophylaxis against group B *Streptococcus*, magnesium sulfate for fetal neuroprotection, antenatal corticosteroids for fetal lung maturity, latency antibiotics for preterm premature rupture of membranes, and tocolysis to allow corticosteroid administration and transfer to a tertiary care center.
- Varying fetal, neonatal, and maternal risks and benefits affect the recommended interventions at a given gestational age.
- Expert opinion and consensus guide preterm delivery management at periviability and the late preterm period, because data are limited.

INTRODUCTION

Preterm birth (birth occurring between 20 0/7 and 36 6/7 weeks' gestation) is the leading cause of neonatal mortality worldwide, with an estimated 14.84 million births, comprising 10.6% of all live births in 2014, increased from 12.9 million (9.6%) in 2005.[1,2] Medically indicated preterm deliveries, multiple gestations, and in vitro fertilization have driven this increase.[3,4]

[a] Division of Maternal Fetal Medicine, Department of Obstetrics and Gynecology, Columbia University Irving Medical Center, 622 East 168th Street PH 16-66, New York, NY 10032, USA;
[b] Department of Obstetrics and Gynecology, Columbia University Irving Medical Center, 622 East 168th Street PH 16-66, New York, NY 10032, USA
* Corresponding author.
E-mail address: js4596@cumc.columbia.edu
Twitter: @MissUkachi (U.N.E.)

Clin Perinatol 47 (2020) 685–703
https://doi.org/10.1016/j.clp.2020.08.006
0095-5108/20/© 2020 Elsevier Inc. All rights reserved.
perinatology.theclinics.com

Most preterm babies survive but face significant short-term and long-term morbidity with increased risk of neurodevelopmental, respiratory, and gastrointestinal issues.[1,4] Preterm births disproportionately account for 75% of all perinatal mortality and more than half of long-term morbidity,[4] with a large contribution from evolving gestational limits of periviability. Increasing survival at earlier gestational ages results in long-term health concerns, including neurologic disability, blindness, deafness, and chronic respiratory disease, which are more likely to be seen in neonates born before 32 weeks or with a birthweight less than 1500 g.[5–7] The treatments that improve premature delivery outcomes target specific morbidities: cerebral palsy, neonatal infection, and fetal lung immaturity.

This article reviews preterm birth interventions intended to reduce neonatal morbidity, examines the existing evidence in preterm birth management, and summarizes the current recommendations for decreasing preterm morbidity and mortality. Specifically, it addresses group B *Streptococcus* (GBS) prophylaxis, magnesium sulfate for neuroprotection, steroids for fetal lung maturity, latency antibiotics for preterm premature rupture of membranes (PPROM), and tocolysis (**Table 1**).

HISTORICAL PERSPECTIVE AND CURRENT EVIDENCE
Group B Streptococcus Prophylaxis

In the 1970s, GBS emerged as one of the leading causes of neonatal morbidity and mortality, with case fatality rates up to 44%. [8,9] The timing of invasive disease represents 2 distinct clinical syndromes, early-onset and late-onset:

- Early-onset disease:
  - Within 7 days of birth
  - Antenatal vertical transmission and/or fetal or neonatal aspiration during labor and delivery
  - Neonatal sepsis, pneumonia, meningitis
- Late-onset disease:
  - Seven days to up to 2 to 3 months after birth
  - Horizontal transmission or nosocomial infection
  - Bacteremia, meningitis, organ and soft tissue infection[8]

Historically, the mortality rates of early-onset disease were significantly higher than those of late-onset disease (55% vs 23%, respectively).[9,10] Intervention is targeted at early-onset GBS disease because it remains the most common cause of early-onset neonatal sepsis.[8]

Maternal vaginal and rectal colonization was identified as the reservoir for vertical transmission.[8,11] Because penicillins for treatment of both GBS urinary tract infections and endometritis decreased colonization rates,[12] maternal prenatal, maternal intrapartum, and neonatal postnatal chemoprophylaxis were investigated to prevent GBS neonatal disease. In a prospective analysis of 32,384 live births between 1973 and 1981, Boyer and colleagues[11] aimed to identify the timing of and risk factors for GBS early-onset disease. Of 61 infants who developed GBS early-onset disease, 65% were bacteremic within 1 hour of life. Despite early postnatal antibiotic treatment, many died, suggesting in utero pathogenesis. These results were supported by several studies estimating the attack rates of GBS early-onset disease based on maternal colonization status at parturition.[9–11] Prospective studies showed only temporary eradication of GBS colonization after antibiotic treatment discontinuation, thus chemoprophylaxis through labor is necessary to suppress maternal and neonatal carriage at birth.[11]

Table 1
Summary of pharmacologic preterm delivery interventions

Intervention	Medication	Dosing	Data	Evidence Type
Prevention of Group B Streptococcus Sepsis	Penicillin G	5 million units IV followed by 2.5–3 million units IV every 4 h until delivery	Tuppurainen and Hallman,[86] 1989	Randomized Controlled Trial
Fetal Lung Maturity	Betamethasone	12 mg IM q24h x 2 doses	Roberts and Dalziel,[87] 2006	Cochrane Review
	Dexamethasone	6mg IM q12h x 4 doses	Brownfoot, et al,[88] 2013	Cochrane Review
Fetal Neuroprotection	Magnesium sulfate	6g IV bolus followed by 2g IV per hour, max 12 h	BEAM Trial Rouse, et al,[28] 2008	Randomized Controlled trial
	Magnesium sulfate	4g IV bolus followed by 1g IV per hour, max 24 h	ACTOMgSO4 Trial Crowther, et al,[25] 2003	Randomized Controlled Trial
	Magnesium sulfate	4g IV bolus, no maintenance	PREMAG Trial Marret, et al,[26,27] 2008	Randomized Controlled Trial
Prolongation of PPROM Latency	Azithromycin PLUS Ampicillin FOLLOWED BY Amoxicillin	1 g PO 2 g IV every 6 h for 48 h 875 mg PO every 12 h OR 500 mg PO every 8 h for an additional 5 d	Kenyon, Boulvain, and Neilson,[44] 2013	Cochrane Review
	Erythromycin PLUS Ampicillin FOLLOWED BY Erythromycin PLUS Amoxicillin	250 mg PO every 8 h for 48 h 2 g IV every 6 h for 48 h 333 mg PO every 8 h 875 mg PO every 12 h OR 500 mg PO every 8 h for an additional 5 d	Mercer, et al,[89,90]	Randomized Controlled Trial Secondary analysis of randomized controlled trial
Uterine Tocolysis for Corticosteroid Completion and/or Maternal Transfer	Nifedipine	20–30 mg PO followed by 10–20 mg every 3–8 h, max 48 h	Flenady, et al,[91] 2014	Cochrane Review
	Inodmethacin	50–100 mg loading dose PO or PR followed by 25 mg P:O every 4–6 h	Reinebrant, et al,[92] 2015	Cochrane Review

Birth weights also affect neonatal GBS illness. Boyer and colleagues[11] showed that both attack rates and case fatality rates increased significantly with birth weights less than 2500 g. Preterm infants have increased morbidity and mortality from GBS disease, likely caused by lower birth weights and increased susceptibility or exposure to infected amniotic fluid.[11,13] Consequently, using intrapartum antibiotic prophylaxis for suppressing maternal GBS colonization became standard of care, with a greater than 80% reduction in GBS early-onset disease incidence,[8] reducing neonatal morbidity and mortality.

Magnesium Sulfate for Fetal Neuroprotection

The tremendous medical advancements improving preterm infant survival have also significantly increased neonatal morbidity, largely from cerebral palsy.[14,15] In the 1980s, very-low-birthweight (VLBW) infants (<1500 g) made up less than 1% of survivors but contributed to 28% of children with disabling cerebral palsy.[16] The high cerebral palsy rate in VLBW infants has been linked to the increased incidence of germinal matrix and intraventricular hemorrhage in this population.[17] Interestingly, multiple prospective trials discovered a decreased neonatal cerebral hemorrhage risk in patients both with preeclampsia and with preterm labor.[18–20] Subsequent observational trials directly linked prenatal exposure to magnesium sulfate with fewer postnatal neurologic morbidities,[20–23] suggesting magnesium sulfate to be neuroprotective for VLBW infants.

Conflicting observational trials led to a series of randomized controlled trials (RCTs) evaluating magnesium sulfate for fetal neuroprotection. Results were summarized in a 2009 Cochrane meta-analysis by Doyle and colleagues,[15] which showed up to a 32% reduction in the risk of cerebral palsy with prenatal magnesium sulfate exposure.[21] Five placebo-controlled RCTs were included in the meta-analysis:

- The Magnesium and Neurologic Endpoints Trial (MagNET, 2002) used magnesium sulfate for preterm labor tocolysis[24]
  - Women less than 34 weeks' gestation
  - Studied rates of cerebral palsy secondarily
- Three RCTs used magnesium sulfate specifically for neuroprotection[25–28]
  - Australasian Collaborative Trial of Magnesium Sulphate (ACTOMgSO4, 2003): women less than 30 weeks' gestation[25]
  - Magnesium Sulphate Given Before Very-preterm Birth to Protect Infant Brain (PREMAG, 2006): women less than 33 weeks' gestation[26,27]
  - Beneficial Effects of Antenatal Magnesium Sulfate (BEAM, 2008): women less than 32 weeks' gestation[28]
- Magnesium Sulphate for the Prevention of Eclampsia (Magpie, 2007) used magnesium sulfate to prevent eclampsia[29]
  - Included pregnancy data up to 37 weeks' gestation
  - Showed no clear difference in death or disability in children at age 18 months, regardless of gestational age at administration

These data and subsequent meta-analyses confirmed the neuroprotective benefits of intravenously administered magnesium sulfate.[15,30] Based on the randomization criteria of the largest trial, BEAM, magnesium sulfate is recommended for fetal neuroprotection for women at imminent risk of delivery before 32 weeks' gestation.

Betamethasone for Fetal Lung Maturity

Respiratory distress syndrome (RDS) has long been acknowledged as a key cause of immediate-term and long-term neonatal morbidity and mortality, but standardized corticosteroid use for promoting fetal lung maturation took decades. As early as 1969, animal studies showed the benefits of antenatal corticosteroids in reducing prematurity-associated morbidity. Liggins[31] observed that the lungs of premature fetal lambs whose mothers were injected with corticosteroids maintained partial lung expansion, unlike those of control premature fetal lambs, which showed alveolar collapse. Subsequently, Crowley and colleagues[32] summarized several human RCTs in a meta-analysis showing that maternal administration of glucocorticoids reduced neonatal RDS, periventricular hemorrhage, necrotizing enterocolitis, and mortality, estimating an odds ratio (OR) of 0.53 (95% confidence interval [CI], 0.44–0.63) for RDS, 0.5 (95% CI, 0.3–0.9) for intraventricular hemorrhage (IVH), and 0.6 (95% CI, 0.48–0.75) for neonatal mortality.[33] Despite this compelling evidence, uncertainty about the efficacy and adverse effects in specific clinical situations (eg, PPROM, diabetes, multifetal gestations) limited corticosteroid use in most preterm deliveries.

To address the discrepancy between antenatal corticosteroid utility and concern for adverse effects, the National Institutes of Health convened for a Consensus Development Conference in 1994. The conference made a clear recommendation for antenatal corticosteroid administration to patients between 24 and 34 weeks' gestation at risk of preterm delivery, with robust evidence for infants born between 29 and 34 weeks.[34] Although no reduction in RDS incidence was seen in infants born between 24 and 28 weeks' gestation, there was a reduction in RDS severity and IVH and mortality incidences. A well-designed retrospective cohort study decades later suggested benefit in multiple gestations between 24 and 33 6/7 weeks, reducing neonatal mortality and short-term respiratory and severe neurologic morbidity, comparable with singletons.[35]

Two subsequent large randomized trials showed a reduction in morbidity in infants born between 34 and 36 6/7 weeks after antenatal corticosteroid administration in the late preterm period:

- Antenatal Steroids for Term Elective Caesarean Section (ASTECS, 2005)[36]
  ○ Betamethasone given within 48 hours before planned 37-week delivery
  ○ Significant reduction in neonatal intensive care unit (NICU) admission for respiratory distress (relative risk, 0.46; 95% CI, 0.23–0.93).
- Antenatal Late Preterm Steroids (ALPS, 2016)[37]
  ○ Betamethasone given to women at risk of late preterm delivery from 34 to 36 6/7 weeks.
  ○ Decreased respiratory support needs within 72 hours after birth, shorter NICU stays, and shorter times until the first feeding, with a small increase neonatal hypoglycemia rates
  ○ No evidence of increased adverse maternal complications
  ○ Patients with PPROM, multiples, a prior steroid course, term cesarean delivery, and pregestational diabetes were excluded

Because antenatal corticosteroid therapy seemed to have the greatest benefit for infants born between 24 hours and 7 days after use,[34] repeat corticosteroid courses became of interest. In the early 2000s, studies of weekly betamethasone showed the marginal benefit of decreased composite morbidity and RDS but revealed conflicting results about adverse effects, particularly intrauterine growth restriction, decreased head circumference, and adverse long-term developmental outcomes not shown in babies exposed to a single antenatal corticosteroid course.[38]

From 2003 to 2008, Garite and colleagues[39] conducted an RCT investigating whether a single rescue course of antenatal corticosteroid therapy could confer benefits without the potential harms seen in multiple repetitive and high-dose courses. Of note, patients with PPROM were excluded, because prior studies showed increased maternal and neonatal infectious morbidity with a second antenatal corticosteroid course.[40,41] Improved neonatal outcomes were shown without increased short-term risk. McEnvoy and colleagues[42] in 2010 showed increased respiratory compliance in infants treated with a single rescue steroid dose. All of these studies used betamethasone and excluded gestations more than 34 weeks. Thus, the American College of Obstetricians and Gynecologists (ACOG) recommends a single repeat corticosteroid dose for women less than 34 weeks' gestation with concern for delivery within 7 days and whose initial course was at least 14 days prior. The rescue course may be administered as early as 7 days after the initial course, if clinically indicated.[43] There is insufficient evidence for rescue steroid use in PPROM.

Antibiotics for Preterm Premature Rupture of Membranes Latency

Approximately one-third of preterm births is associated with PPROM, thought to be caused predominantly by inflammation and infection.[44,45] Antibiotic use attempts to prolong latency after PPROM. In 1963, Lebherz and colleagues[46] studied antibiotic therapy for PPROM, using demethylchlortetracycline, which was ultimately shown to be teratogenic. In the late 1980s and 1990s, ampicillin was trialed to decrease maternal and perinatal morbidity from transplacental and genital tract passage of pathogens such as GBS, the viridans group *streptococci*, *Escherichia coli*, and *Haemophilus influenzae*.[47] Morbidities included neonatal sepsis, neonatal complications of prematurity (eg, RDS, IVH, necrotizing enterocolitis), chorioamnionitis, and endometritis. The prolonged latency period between the PPROM occurrence and delivery was consistently observed and has become one of the primary objectives of prophylactic antibiotic administration, along with reducing other causes of perinatal and maternal morbidity.[47,48]

Amniotic fluid and placental cultures implicated anaerobic bacteria in PPROM pathogenesis, informing modern latency antibiotic regimens to including a macrolide antibiotic for broader-spectrum coverage.[49] A 2013 Cochrane Review of 22 placebo-controlled randomized trials from 1988 to 2006 involving 6872 women delivering at less than 37 weeks' gestation and their infants concluded that antibiotics following PPROM significantly reduce chorioamnionitis and progression to delivery within 48 hours and within 7 days.[44] It also showed decreased neonatal morbidity, including neonatal infections, surfactant use, need for oxygen therapy, and abnormal cerebral ultrasonography findings before discharge. However, because amoxicillin-clavulanic acid resulted in an increased neonatal necrotizing enterocolitis risk, alternate regimens should be considered. In addition, neonatal benefits of expectant management between 34 and 36 6/7 weeks' gestation are marginal, compared with the significant risks of maternal morbidity.[50] Although expectant management can be considered in this late preterm phase, latency antibiotics are deemed not appropriate. The recommended prophylactic antibiotic combinations for PPROM have been determined by expert opinion and committee recommendations to standardize practice.[51]

Tocolysis

Because preterm labor precedes 40% to 50% of preterm deliveries, tocolytic medications (eg, betamimetic agents, magnesium sulfate, calcium channel blockers, and prostaglandin synthase inhibitors) have been used to inhibit myometrial contractions in attempts to prevent preterm birth and its associated morbidity and mortality.[4,52] Although they have not significantly reduced preterm birth rates, tocolytics aid other interventions that reduce neonatal morbidity, such as antenatal corticosteroids.

In the 1950s and 1960s, fetal maturity was noted to be a significant predictor of morbidity independent of neonatal size. In 1950, the World Health Organization (WHO) defined prematurity by birthweight ($\leq$2500 g), but redefined it by gestational age (<37 weeks) in 1962.[52] In 1955, tocolysis was first attempted using the protein relaxin, known to cause uterine relaxation,[53] which was followed by ethanol, introduced by Fuchs and colleagues[54] in 1967 for its inhibitory effect on oxytocin release. Because relaxin did not show efficacy in subsequent trials, and the effective doses of ethanol caused adverse maternal and fetal effects, both agents have been abandoned in modern obstetric practice.

Magnesium sulfate showed early promise as a tocolytic agent in the late 1950s and 1960s, based on the incidental finding of prolonging labor when used for preeclampsia management.[55] Laboratory experiments showed it impaired myometrial contractility.[56] Because the original promising trials were flawed, systematic reviews of subsequent RCTs were conducted by Cochrane, by an independent review from Canada, and by the US Agency for Healthcare Research and Quality.[57–59] These reviews all concluded that magnesium sulfate does not reduce the risk of preterm delivery compared with placebo but does increase the risk of adverse outcomes (eg, fetal and neonatal death) because of the high doses required for tocolytic effect.[59]

The tocolytic agents successful in clinical trials and modern practice are betamimetics (beta-agonists), calcium channel blockers, and prostaglandin synthetase inhibitors. A detailed description of each is presented in **Table 2**. The evidence for their efficacy is as follows:

- Betamimetics
  - RCTs show they reduce the risk of delivery within 48 hours, an effect even greater at 24 hours[60]
  - One early study showed up to a 7-day delay in delivery, but no consistent reduction in preterm delivery rate[61]
  - Maternal cardiopulmonary and metabolic side effects have limited the use of beta-agonists for tocolysis[60]
- Calcium channel blockers
  - Nifedipine reduced uterine activity in nonpregnant patients with primary dysmenorrhea and pregnant patients undergoing therapeutic abortions, thus was studied as a tocolytic in 1980 to allow corticosteroid administration before delivery[62]
  - In RCTs, nifedipine consistently delayed delivery up to 48 hours and up to 1 week
  - Efficacy similar to or greater than betamimetics with a more favorable side effect profile[60]
- Prostaglandin synthetase inhibitors
  - Play a role in labor physiology and preterm labor pathophysiology
  - 1972: Indomethacin inhibited spontaneous contractions in rat uteri in vitro[48]
  - 1974: Indomethacin stopped contractions in 80% of women in preterm labor[63]
  - Ketorolac and sulindac reduced the rate of delivery within 48 hours in RCTs[60]
  - Overall well tolerated by patients, but should be avoided in several maternal conditions
  - Indomethacin crosses the placenta, with potentially critical fetal side effects[60]
    - Observational studies and secondary data analyses showed prostaglandin synthetase inhibitors used for longer than 72 hours cause constriction and premature closure of the ductus arteriosus or primary pulmonary hypertension
    - Association even more striking in fetuses more than 32 weeks' gestation, suggesting increased sensitivity of the ductus arteriosus to the agents after this period

Table 2
Pharmacologic and clinical characteristics of efficacious tocolytic agents[60]

Class	Mechanism	Example Agents	Contraindications	Maternal Side Effects	Fetal Side Effects
Betamimetics (Beta-agonists)	Inhibit muscle contraction: act on the β2 uterine smooth muscle cell receptors → increase cyclic adenosine monophosphate → decreasing free calcium and phosphorylating myosin light-chain kinase	Terbutaline[a] Ritodrine Albuterol Fenoterol Hexoprenaline Isoxsuprine Metaproterenol Nylidrin Orciprenaline Salbutamol	• Cardiac arrhythmias • Poorly controlled thyrotoxicosis • Poorly controlled diabetes mellitus	• Tachyphylaxis • Cardiopulmonary (tachycardia, hypotension, arrhythmias, myocardial ischemia, pulmonary edema) • Metabolic (hyperglycemia, hypokalemia)	• Cardiac (tachycardia) • Metabolic (hypoglycemia, hyperbilirubinemia and hypocalcemia)
Calcium channel blockers	Decrease myometrial activity: reduce intracellular calcium → inhibit myosin light-chain kinase phosphorylation, reduce uterine vascular resistance	Nifedipine[a] Nicardipine	• Maternal hypotension • Concomitant magnesium sulfate use (reports of neuromuscular blockade)	• Transient hypotension • Minor symptoms (flushing, dizziness, headache, nausea	None shown to date

| Prostaglandin synthetase inhibitors | Decrease contractile activity: inhibit cyclooxygenase → decrease prostaglandin synthetase, block conversion of free arachidonic acid to prostaglandin (mediator of uterine contractions) | Indomethacin[a] Ketorolac Sulindac[b] | • Significant hepatic or renal impairment
• Active peptic ulcer disease
• NSAID sensitivity, NSAID-sensitive asthma
• Coagulation disorders, thrombocytopenia
• Careful consideration in cases of oligohydramnios | • Minor symptoms (nausea, heartburn) | Most reported with prolonged use, large doses, use after 32 wk
• Premature constriction of the ductus arteriosus (resultant pulmonary hypertension)
• Reversible decrease in renal function (resultant oligohydramnios)
• IVH, NEC, hyperbilirubinemia |

Abbreviations: NEC, necrotizing enterocolitis; NSAID, nonsteroidal antiinflammatory drug.

[a] Commonly used for tocolysis in the Unites States. Though ritodrine was the only betamimetic that was FDA-approved for use in preterm labor, it has since been removed from the market because of concern for serious adverse maternal effects.

[b] Less potent maternal and fetal adverse effects compared with other prostaglandin synthetase inhibitors.

Data from Hearne AE, Nagey DA. Therapeutic agents in preterm labor: tocolytic agents. Clin Obstet Gynecol. 2000;43(4):787-801.

○ Other potential fetal effects are listed in **Table 2**

A tocolytic agent should meet 3 criteria: (1) delays labor, (2) safe for mother and fetus, and (3) improves perinatal outcomes.[64] Betamimetics, calcium channel blockers, and prostaglandin synthetase inhibitors all delay labor at least 48 hours, and in some cases up to 7 days. They are generally safe. However, RCTs have not shown improvements in neonatal outcomes or consistent increases in mean delivery gestational age with prolonged or recurrent tocolytic use.[60,65] At present, tocolytics are recommended for delaying birth for the 24 to 48 hours necessary to transfer the patient to a tertiary care center and/or to administer corticosteroids for fetal lung maturity, both clearly improving neonatal outcomes.[52] Similarly, insufficient evidence exists for tocolysis for PPROM, because it increases chorioamnionitis without significant neonatal benefit.[66] However, the patients in the systematic review did not routinely receive latency antibiotics or betamethasone, which are now standards of care.

The use of tocolytics is controversial, with suspected placental abruption. A few retrospective cohort studies have shown potential benefit without harm in select cases where the fetal status seems reassuring and the patient is medically stable.[67–69] However, no prospective studies support this use, even with clinically stable patients.

MANAGEMENT RECOMMENDATIONS BY GESTATIONAL AGE

Preterm birth management varies by gestational age because of the increasing perinatal morbidity with decreasing gestational age:

- Periviable: 20 to 25 6/7 weeks
- Extremely preterm: less than 28 weeks
- Very preterm: 28 to 31 6/7 weeks
- Moderately preterm: 32 to 33 6/7 weeks
- Late preterm: 34 to 36 6/7 weeks

Clinical management recommendations change as the risks and benefits shift with each gestational age group. Recommended interventions by gestational age are summarized in **Fig. 1**.

Special Considerations: Periviability

Before 1980, infants born at or before 24 weeks' gestation, regardless of birth weight, were not expected to survive.[70] Despite progressively increasing survival rates of infants born at 22 to 25 weeks' gestation, most have neurodevelopmental concerns.[71] Between 2001 and 2011, Younge and colleagues[72] performed an 11-center study reviewing survival and neurologic outcomes of more than 4000 deliveries between 22 and 24 weeks' gestation, finding an increase in overall survival rate and survival without neurodevelopmental impairment. However, mortalities of 97% to 98% were seen in infants born between 22 0/7 and 22 6/7 weeks, with only 1% surviving neurologically intact.[72] Neurodevelopmental outcomes improved with increasing gestational age, with 55% of infants born between 24 0/7 and 24 6/7 weeks' gestation surviving, and 32% surviving without evidence of neurodevelopmental impairment at 18 to 22 months' corrected age.[72]

Because of increased neonatal survival rates in earlier gestational ages, the term periviable birth (delivery occurring from 20 0/7 to 25 6/7 weeks' gestation) was coined in a joint workshop of the Society for Maternal-Fetal Medicine (SMFM), the *Eunice Kennedy Shriver* National Institute of Child Health and Human Development (NICHD), the Section on Perinatal Pediatrics, and ACOG.[73] Treatment recommendations combine data extrapolated from older gestational ages and expert opinion, because

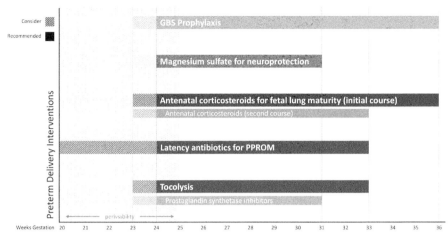

Fig. 1. Considerations and recommendations for preterm delivery interventions by gestational age. The recommendations for intervention include the entire week of gestation on which the bar terminates; for example, magnesium sulfate is recommended through the 31st week of gestation up until and including 31 6/7.

of the lack of studies including gestations before 24 weeks. However, prospective data on antenatal corticosteroids in the periviable period do exist. A NICHD prospective cohort study of 10,541 infants born at 22 to 25 weeks' gestation showed reductions in death and neurodevelopmental impairment at 18 to 22 months for those exposed to antenatal corticosteroids born at 23, 24, and 25 weeks. There was no outcome difference at 22 weeks' gestation.[74] Without capability for neonatal resuscitation (ie, 20–22 6/7 weeks' gestation in most institutions), morbidity-reducing interventions such as tocolysis and antenatal corticosteroids are not recommended. However, unlike other interventions discussed in this article, latency antibiotics for PPROM have a role outside of reduction of morbidity and therefore should be considered during the entire periviable period if delivery is not imminent.[71]

Shared decision making regarding preterm birth interventions in the periviable period should involve the NICU team and consider maternal and neonatal risks, parental preferences, and the gestational age after which neonatal resuscitation is obligatory (typically 24 weeks, although this may be location dependent), because periviable infants do not survive without life-sustaining interventions. The discussion should include goals of care (eg, optimizing survival or minimizing suffering) as well as institution-specific outcomes. Advancements in treatments and resuscitation capabilities at tertiary care centers have now shifted the limits of viability to earlier gestational ages, with some centers offering the initiation of resuscitation as early as 22 to 23 weeks, but with severe neurodevelopmental impairment.

Special Considerations: Maternal Health Implications of Cesarean Delivery for Fetal Indication

Preterm birth has significant implications for maternal health and neonatal outcomes. One study of 2659 women delivering between 23 and 33 weeks' gestation found composite complication rates of 8.6%, including hemorrhage, infection, ICU admission, and death.[75] Complication frequency was associated with both gestational age and delivery route, being highest between 23 and 27 weeks' gestation and with classic cesarean, respectively.[75] If a cesarean is medically necessary, earlier gestational ages result in a higher likelihood of a classical hysterotomy (vertical uterine incision extending to the upper muscular portion of the uterus) and other associated morbidities.

A study by Bertholdt and colleagues[76] compared cesarean deliveries between 24 to 25 and 26 to 27 weeks' gestation, noting higher composite intraoperative complications in the former (63.5% vs 30.8%; adjusted OR, 5.04):

- Classical hysterotomy
- Transplacental delivery
- Difficult fetal extraction
- Postpartum hemorrhage
- Internal organ injury

Besides being associated with more frequent perioperative morbidities than a low transverse uterine incision in the index delivery, a Classical hysterotomy leads to an increased risk of uterine rupture in subsequent pregnancies, thus repeat cesareans are required for all future deliveries. The future reproductive risks associated with cesarean delivery increase with each subsequent cesarean.[71] Lannon and colleagues[77] showed that, regardless of incision type, periviable cesareans increase uterine rupture risk by 1.8% in subsequent pregnancies, going up to 2.5% in women with a prior classic incision.

A history of a prior cesarean also significantly increases the risk for abnormal placentation, including placenta previa and placenta accreta spectrum disorder, which may lead to cesarean hysterectomy.[78] The past 4 decades have seen a higher number of patients with abnormal placentation, mostly caused by increased cesarean rates.[78] Maternal morbidity and mortality risk with placenta accreta spectrum is increased because of the possibility of severe hemorrhage and intraoperative and postoperative complications.

Few data suggest that classic cesarean for malpresentation in periviable gestations, where the greatest maternal morbidity lies, improves long-term outcomes. In a retrospective cohort of pregnancies with breech fetuses at 23 to 24 weeks' gestation, cesarean-born infants had overall improved survival (adjusted OR, 2.91), but intubated neonates showed no survival difference up to more than 6 months' corrected age, despite the short-term survival advantage.[79] Given the increased morbidity at earlier gestational ages without clear neonatal advantage, cesarean before 22 weeks' gestation is appropriate only for maternal indications.[71]

DISCUSSION

Preterm infant outcomes have improved over the last several decades because of advancements in preterm and postnatal treatments.[80] GBS prophylaxis, magnesium sulfate, antenatal corticosteroids, latency antibiotics for PPROM, and tocolysis through the antenatal corticosteroid window and during transfer to tertiary care centers represent the best interventions currently available to improve preterm neonatal outcomes. The evidence discussed earlier suggests:

- Antibiotics for GBS suppression reduce early-onset neonatal sepsis and neonatal morbidity and mortality
- Magnesium sulfate reduces cerebral palsy and gross motor dysfunction risks
- Antenatal corticosteroids reduce respiratory distress and fetal and neonatal deaths
- Latency antibiotics for PPROM reduce chorioamnionitis and increase duration from membrane rupture to delivery, increasing the gestational age at birth and decreasing neonatal morbidity

- Tocolytics allow time for transfer to a tertiary care center and for administration of other recommended pharmacologic interventions

Pharmacologic interventions should be offered to all women at risk of preterm birth unless otherwise contraindicated. Treatments vary by gestational age: all interventions are recommended for extremely preterm and very preterm fetuses, all except magnesium sulfate are recommended for moderate preterm fetuses, and only GBS prophylaxis and a single course of antenatal corticosteroids (if steroid naive) are recommended in the late preterm period, affirmed by ACOG, SMFM, and WHO, among others.[51,81,82]

The pharmacologic interventions listed earlier have been discussed individually but are used concordantly in practice; the impact of simultaneous interventions on outcomes is an important future research direction. Prospective observational studies of extremely preterm infants show concordant use of both antenatal corticosteroids and magnesium sulfate improves neonatal outcomes more than antenatal corticosteroid use alone.[83] Additional investigations of a wider gestational age range could show the effect of multiple concurrent pharmacologic interventions on outcomes, although studies may be difficult to perform because these interventions are already the standard of practice.

All preterm birth interventions are contingent on accurately identifying the women who will ultimately deliver preterm, because preterm labor can spontaneously resolve. Approximately half of women hospitalized for preterm labor give birth at term.[84] The early identification of at-risk women may depend on access to prenatal care and use of diagnostic evaluations such as cervical length measurements and testing for fetal fibronectin. Once women are identified to be at risk for preterm labor, pharmacologic interventions should be prompt. Identification of at-risk women for indicated preterm birth is less challenging, because maternal, fetal, and placental conditions (eg, hypertension, diabetes mellitus, and intrauterine growth restriction) necessitating preterm delivery often require frequent monitoring. Swift pharmacologic intervention is essential for indicated preterm birth, particularly because of the higher neonatal morbidity risk compared with spontaneous preterm birth.[85]

Reducing neonatal morbidity and mortality from preterm birth requires a multimodal approach across the reproductive timeline, from preconception counseling to prevention measures to delivery interventions and time interval to the next conception. Overall preterm infant survival has improved but the shift in the lower limits of periviability worsens short-term and long-term health implications for both the neonates and the mothers, with delivery at earlier gestational ages portending more risk. Further research into the pathophysiology of preterm birth is imperative for determining strategies for prevention, such as targeting modifiable risk factors, in order to improve outcomes. In the interim, the pharmacologic interventions discussed in this article remain the mainstay of improving neonatal outcomes for preterm deliveries.

Best Practices

What is the current practice?

Preterm delivery interventions
  Best practice/guideline/care path objectives
  - Use of pharmacologic preterm delivery interventions to improve neonatal preterm birth outcomes, including:
    ○ GBS prophylaxis
    ○ Magnesium sulfate for fetal neuroprotection
    ○ Antenatal corticosteroids for fetal lung maturation

- ○ Latency antibiotics for PPROM
- ○ Tocolysis to allow other interventions and/or for transfer to tertiary care center

What changes in current practice are likely to improve outcomes?

- Earlier identification of women at risk of preterm delivery
- Swift implementation of pharmacologic preterm delivery interventions
- Adherence to algorithms regarding use of pharmacologic interventions by gestational age

Major recommendations

Preterm delivery interventions should be used according to gestational age as follows:
- Early periviability 20 0/7 to 23 6/7 weeks
  - ○ Shared decision making regarding neonatal intervention and resuscitation
  - ○ Consider GBS prophylaxis at 23 0/7 weeks (level 2B)
  - ○ Consider magnesium sulfate for fetal neuroprotection at 23 0/7 weeks (level 2B)
  - ○ Consider corticosteroids for fetal lung maturity at 23 0/7 weeks (level 2B)
  - ○ Consider latency antibiotics for PPROM at 20 0/7 weeks (level 2C 20 0/7–22 6/7 weeks, level 2B 23 0/7–23 6/7 weeks)
  - ○ Consider tocolysis for corticosteroid administration at 23 0/7 weeks (level 2B)
- Extremely preterm 24 0/7 to 28 0/7 weeks and very preterm 28 0/7 to 31 6/7 weeks (level 1B)
  - ○ Expectant management if no contraindications
  - ○ GBS prophylaxis
  - ○ Magnesium sulfate for fetal neuroprotection
  - ○ Corticosteroids for fetal lung maturity
  - ○ Second (rescue) course of betamethasone if at imminent risk of delivery
  - ○ Latency antibiotics for PPROM
  - ○ Tocolysis during antenatal corticosteroid course and for transfer to tertiary care center
- Moderate preterm 32 0/7 to 33 6/7 weeks (level 1B)
  - ○ Expectant management if no contraindications
  - ○ GBS prophylaxis
  - ○ Corticosteroids for fetal lung maturity
  - ○ Second (rescue) course of betamethasone if at imminent risk of delivery
  - ○ Latency antibiotics for PPROM
  - ○ Tocolysis during antenatal corticosteroid course and for transfer to tertiary care center
- Late preterm 34 0/7 to 36 6/7 weeks (level 1B)
  - ○ Expectant management if no contraindications
  - ○ GBS prophylaxis
  - ○ Single course of corticosteroids for fetal lung maturity if steroid naive

Summary statement

Early identification of women at risk of preterm delivery and rapid use of pharmacologic preterm delivery interventions are critical in improving preterm neonatal outcomes.

Bibliographic sources: Refs.[8,21,43,51,71,74,81,82]

DISCLOSURE

The authors have nothing to disclose.

CLINICS CARE POINTS

- Antibiotics for Group B Streptococcus suppression reduce early-onset neonatal sepsis and neonatal morbidity and mortality.
- Magnesium sulfate reduces cerebral palsy and gross motor dysfunction risks.
- Antenatal corticosteroids reduce respiratory distress and fetal and neonatal deaths.

- Latency antibiotics for PPROM reduce chorioamnionitis and increase duration from membrane rupture to delivery, increasing the gestational age at birth and decreasing neonatal morbidity.
- Tocolytics allow time for transfer to a tertiary care center and for administration of other recommended pharmacologic interventions.

REFERENCES

1. Chawanpaiboon S, Vogel JP, Moller A-B, et al. Global, regional, and national estimates of levels of preterm birth in 2014: a systematic review and modelling analysis. Lancet Glob Health 2019;7(1):e37–46.
2. Beck S, Wojdyla D, Say L, et al. The worldwide incidence of preterm birth: a systematic review of maternal mortality and morbidity. Bull World Health Organ 2010; 88(1):31–8.
3. Purisch SE, Gyamfi-Bannerman C. Epidemiology of preterm birth. Semin Perinatol 2017;41(7):387–91.
4. Goldenberg RL, Culhane JF, Iams JD, et al. Epidemiology and causes of preterm birth. Lancet 2008;371(9606):75–84.
5. Vohr BR, Wright LL, Poole WK, et al. Neurodevelopmental outcomes of extremely low birth weight infants <32 weeks' gestation between 1993 and 1998. Pediatrics 2005;116(3):635–43.
6. Hack M, Flannery DJ, Schluchter M, et al. Outcomes in young adulthood for very-low-birth-weight infants. N Engl J Med 2002;346(3):149–57.
7. Hintz SR, Kendrick DE, Vohr BR, et al. Changes in neurodevelopmental outcomes at 18 to 22 months' corrected age among infants of less than 25 weeks' gestational age born in 1993-1999. Pediatrics 2005;115(6):1645–51.
8. Prevention of Group B. Streptococcal early-onset disease in newborns: ACOG committee opinion, number 797. Obstet Gynecol 2020;135(2):e51–72.
9. Anthony BF, Okada DM. The emergence of group B streptococci in infections of the newborn infant. Annu Rev Med 1977;28:355–69.
10. Baker CJ. Summary of the workshop on perinatal infections due to group B Streptococcus. J Infect Dis 1977;136(1):137–52.
11. Boyer KM, Gadzala CA, Burd LI, et al. Selective intrapartum chemoprophylaxis of neonatal group B streptococcal early-onset disease. I. Epidemiologic rationale. J Infect Dis 1983;148(5):795–801.
12. Anthony BF, Okada DM, Hobel CJ. Epidemlology of group B Streptococcus: longitudinal observations during pregnancy. J Infect Dis 1978;137(5):524–30.
13. Ancona RJ, Ferrieri P, Williams PP. Maternal factors that enhance the acquisition of group-B streptococci by newborn infants. J Med Microbiol 1980;13(2):273–80.
14. Hirtz DG, Nelson K. Magnesium sulfate and cerebral palsy in premature infants. Curr Opin Pediatr 1998;10(2):131–7.
15. Doyle LW, Crowther CA, Middleton P, et al. Magnesium sulphate for women at risk of preterm birth for neuroprotection of the fetus. Cochrane Database Syst Rev 2009;(1):CD004661.
16. Nelson KB, Grether JK. Can magnesium sulfate reduce the risk of cerebral palsy in very low birthweight infants? Pediatrics 1995;95(2):263–9.
17. Vohr B, Garcia Coll C, Flanagan P, et al. Effects of intraventricular hemorrhage and socioeconomic status on perceptual, cognitive, and neurologic status of low birth weight infants at 5 years of age. J Pediatr 1992;121(2):280–5.

18. van de Bor M, Verloove-Vanhorick SP, Brand R, et al. Incidence and prediction of periventricular-intraventricular hemorrhage in very preterm infants. J Perinat Med 1987;15(4):333–9.

19. Leviton A, Kuban KC, Pagano M, et al. Maternal toxemia and neonatal germinal matrix hemorrhage in intubated infants less than 1751 g. Obstet Gynecol 1988; 72(4):571–6.

20. Kuban KC, Leviton A, Pagano M, et al. Maternal toxemia is associated with reduced incidence of germinal matrix hemorrhage in premature babies. J Child Neurol 1992;7(1):70–6.

21. Committee Opinion No. 455: magnesium sulfate before anticipated preterm birth for neuroprotection. Obstet Gynecol 2010;115(3):669–71.

22. Schendel DE, Berg CJ, Yeargin-Allsopp M, et al. Prenatal magnesium sulfate exposure and the risk for cerebral palsy or mental retardation among very low-birth-weight children aged 3 to 5 years. JAMA 1996;276(22):1805–10.

23. Paneth N, Jetton J, Pinto-Martin J, et al. Magnesium sulfate in labor and risk of neonatal brain lesions and cerebral palsy in low birth weight infants. The Neonatal Brain Hemorrhage Study Analysis Group. Pediatrics 1997;99(5):E1.

24. Mittendorf R, Dambrosia J, Pryde PG, et al. Association between the use of ante-natal magnesium sulfate in preterm labor and adverse health outcomes in infants. Am J Obstet Gynecol 2002;186(6):1111–8.

25. Crowther CA, Hiller JE, Doyle LW, et al. Australasian Collaborative Trial of Magne-sium Sulphate Collaborative G. Effect of magnesium sulfate given for neuropro-tection before preterm birth: a randomized controlled trial. JAMA 2003;290(20): 2669–76.

26. Marret S, Marpeau L, Zupan-Simunek V, et al. Magnesium sulphate given before very-preterm birth to protect infant brain: the randomised controlled PREMAG trial*. BJOG 2007;114(3):310–8.

27. Marret S, Marpeau L, Follet-Bouhamed C, et al. [Effect of magnesium sulphate on mortality and neurologic morbidity of the very-preterm newborn (of less than 33 weeks) with two-year neurological outcome: results of the prospective PRE-MAG trial]. Gynecol Obstet Fertil 2008;36(3):278–88.

28. Rouse DJ, Hirtz DG, Thom E, et al. A randomized, controlled trial of magnesium sulfate for the prevention of cerebral palsy. N Engl J Med 2008;359(9):895–905.

29. Magpie Trial Follow-Up Study Collaborative G. The Magpie Trial: a randomised trial comparing magnesium sulphate with placebo for pre-eclampsia. Outcome for children at 18 months. BJOG 2007;114(3):289–99.

30. Costantine MM, Weiner SJ, Eunice Kennedy Shriver National Institute of Child Health and Human Development Maternal-Fetal Medicine Units Network. Human Development Maternal-Fetal Medicine Units N. Effects of antenatal exposure to magnesium sulfate on neuroprotection and mortality in preterm infants: a meta-analysis. Obstet Gynecol 2009;114(2 Pt 1):354–64.

31. Liggins GC. Premature delivery of foetal lambs infused with glucocorticoids. J Endocrinol 1969;45(4):515–23.

32. Crowley PA. Antenatal corticosteroid therapy: a meta-analysis of the randomized trials, 1972 to 1994. Am J Obstet Gynecol 1995;173(1):322–35.

33. Di Renzo GC, Roura LC, European Association of Perinatal Medicine-Study Group on Preterm Birth. Guidelines for the management of spontaneous preterm labor. J Perinat Med 2006;34(5):359–66.

34. Effect of corticosteroids for fetal maturation on perinatal outcomes. NIH Consens Statement 1994;12(2):1–24.

35. Melamed N, Shah J, Yoon EW, et al. The role of antenatal corticosteroids in twin pregnancies complicated by preterm birth. Am J Obstet Gynecol 2016;215(4): 482.e1-9.

36. Stutchfield P, Whitaker R, Russell I. Antenatal Steroids for Term Elective Caesarean Section Research T. Antenatal betamethasone and incidence of neonatal respiratory distress after elective caesarean section: pragmatic randomised trial. BMJ 2005;331(7518):662.

37. Gyamfi-Bannerman C, Thom EA. Antenatal betamethasone for women at risk for late preterm delivery. N Engl J Med 2016;375(5):486-7.

38. Crowther CA, McKinlay CJ, Middleton P, et al. Repeat doses of prenatal corticosteroids for women at risk of preterm birth for improving neonatal health outcomes. Cochrane Database Syst Rev 2015;(7):CD003935.

39. Garite TJ, Kurtzman J, Maurel K, et al. Impact of a 'rescue course' of antenatal corticosteroids: a multicenter randomized placebo-controlled trial. Am J Obstet Gynecol 2009;200(3):248.e1-9.

40. Vermillion ST, Soper DE, Chasedunn-Roark J. Neonatal sepsis after betamethasone administration to patients with preterm premature rupture of membranes. Am J Obstet Gynecol 1999;181(2):320-7.

41. Lee MJ, Davies J, Guinn D, et al. Single versus weekly courses of antenatal corticosteroids in preterm premature rupture of membranes. Obstet Gynecol 2004; 103(2):274-81.

42. McEvoy C, Schilling D, Peters D, et al. Respiratory compliance in preterm infants after a single rescue course of antenatal steroids: a randomized controlled trial. Am J Obstet Gynecol 2010;202(6):544.e1-9.

43. Antenatal corticosteroid therapy for fetal maturation. Committee Opinion No. 713. American College of Obstetricians and Gynecologists. Obstet Gynecol 2017;130: e102-9.

44. Kenyon S, Boulvain M, Neilson JP. Antibiotics for preterm rupture of membranes. Cochrane Database Syst Rev 2013;(12):CD001058.

45. Bejar R, Curbelo V, Davis C, et al. Premature labor. II. Bacterial sources of phospholipase. Obstet Gynecol 1981;57(4):479-82.

46. Lebherz TB, Hellman LP, Madding R, et al. Double-Blind study of premature rupture of the membranes. A report of 1,896 cases. Am J Obstet Gynecol 1963;87:218-25.

47. Greenberg RT, Hankins GD. Antibiotic therapy in preterm premature rupture of membranes. Clin Obstet Gynecol 1991;34(4):742-50.

48. Vane JR, Williams KI. Prostaglandin production contributes to the contractions of the rat isolated uterus. Br J Pharmacol 1972;45(1):146P.

49. Lewis DF, Fontenot MT, Brooks GG, et al. Latency period after preterm premature rupture of membranes: a comparison of ampicillin with and without sulbactam. Obstet Gynecol 1995;86(3):392-5.

50. Prelabor rupture of membranes: ACOG practice bulletin, number 217. Obstet Gynecol 2020;135(3):e80-97.

51. SMFM PTB Toolkit Task Force. SMFM preterm birth toolkit. Society for Maternal-Fetal Medicine. 2016. Available at: https://www.smfm.org/publications/231-smfm-preterm-birth-toolkit. Accessed May 16, 2020.

52. Keirse MJ. The history of tocolysis. BJOG 2003;110(Suppl 20):94-7.

53. Abramson D, Reid DE. Use of relaxin in treatment of threatened premature labor. J Clin Endocrinol Metab 1955;15(2):206-9.

54. Fuchs F, Fuchs AR, Poblete VF Jr, et al. Effect of alcohol on threatened premature labor. Am J Obstet Gynecol 1967;99(5):627-37.

55. Hall DG, Mc GH Jr, Corey EL, et al. The effects of magnesium therapy on the duration of labor. Am J Obstet Gynecol 1959;78(1):27–32.
56. Mittendorf R, Pryde PG. A review of the role for magnesium sulphate in preterm labour. BJOG 2005;112(Suppl 1):84–8.
57. Crowther CA, Hiller JE, Doyle LW. Magnesium sulphate for preventing preterm birth in threatened preterm labour. Cochrane Database Syst Rev 2002;(4):CD001060.
58. Gyetvai K, Hannah ME, Hodnett ED, et al. Tocolytics for preterm labor: a systematic review. Obstet Gynecol 1999;94(5 Pt 2):869–77.
59. Grimes DA, Nanda K. Magnesium sulfate tocolysis: time to quit. Obstet Gynecol 2006;108(4):986–9.
60. Hearne AE, Nagey DA. Therapeutic agents in preterm labor: tocolytic agents. Clin Obstet Gynecol 2000;43(4):787–801.
61. Wesselius-de Casparis A, Thiery M, Yo le Sian A, et al. Results of double-blind, multicentre study with ritodrine in premature labour. Br Med J 1971;3(5767):144–7.
62. Ulmsten U, Andersson KE, Wingerup L. Treatment of premature labor with the calcium antagonist nifedipine. Arch Gynecol 1980;229(1):1–5.
63. Zuckerman H, Reiss U, Rubinstein I. Inhibition of human premature labor by indomethacin. Obstet Gynecol 1974;44(6):787–92.
64. Fisk N. The case for tocolysis in threatened preterm labour. BJOG 2003;110:98–102.
65. Dehaene I, Bergman L, Turtiainen P, et al. Maintaining and repeating tocolysis: a reflection on evidence. Semin Perinatol 2017;41(8):468–76.
66. Mackeen AD, Seibel-Seamon J, Muhammad J, et al. Tocolytics for preterm premature rupture of membranes. Cochrane Database Syst Rev 2014;(2):CD007062.
67. Sholl JS. Abruptio placentae: clinical management in nonacute cases. Am J Obstet Gynecol 1987;156(1):40–51.
68. Saller DN Jr, Nagey DA, Pupkin MJ, et al. Tocolysis in the management of third trimester bleeding. J Perinatol 1990;10(2):125–8.
69. Towers CV, Pircon RA, Heppard M. Is tocolysis safe in the management of third-trimester bleeding? Am J Obstet Gynecol 1999;180(6 Pt 1):1572–8.
70. Koops BL, Morgan LJ, Battaglia FC. Neonatal mortality risk in relation to birth weight and gestational age: update. J Pediatr 1082;101(C).909–77.
71. American College of Obstetricians and Gynecologists, Society for Maternal-Fetal Medicine. Obstetric care consensus No. 6: periviable birth. Obstet Gynecol 2017;130(4):e187–99.
72. Younge N, Goldstein RF, Bann CM, et al. Survival and neurodevelopmental outcomes among periviable infants. N Engl J Med 2017;376(7):617–28.
73. Raju TN, Mercer BM, Burchfield DJ, et al. Periviable birth: executive summary of a joint workshop by the Eunice Kennedy Shriver National Institute of Child Health and Human Development, Society for Maternal-Fetal Medicine, American Academy of Pediatrics, and American College of Obstetricians and Gynecologists. Obstet Gynecol 2014;123(5):1083–96.
74. Carlo WA, McDonald SA, Fanaroff AA, et al. Association of antenatal corticosteroids with mortality and neurodevelopmental outcomes among infants born at 22 to 25 weeks' gestation. JAMA 2011;306(21):2348–58.
75. Reddy UM, Rice MM, Grobman WA, et al. Serious maternal complications after early preterm delivery (24-33 weeks' gestation). Am J Obstet Gynecol 2015;213(4):538.e1-9.

76. Bertholdt C, Menard S, Delorme P, et al. Intraoperative adverse events associ-
    ated with extremely preterm cesarean deliveries. Acta Obstet Gynecol Scand
    2018;97(5):608–14.
77. Lannon SM, Guthrie KA, Vanderhoeven JP, et al. Uterine rupture risk after perivi-
    able cesarean delivery. Obstet Gynecol 2015;125(5):1095–100.
78. Obstetric care consensus No. 7: placenta accreta spectrum. Obstet Gynecol
    2018;132(6):e259–75.
79. Tucker Edmonds B, McKenzie F, Macheras M, et al. Morbidity and mortality asso-
    ciated with mode of delivery for breech periviable deliveries. Am J Obstet Gyne-
    col 2015;213(1):70.e1-12.
80. Iams JD, Romero R, Culhane JF, et al. Primary, secondary, and tertiary interven-
    tions to reduce the morbidity and mortality of preterm birth. Lancet 2008;
    371(9607):164–75.
81. American College of Obstetricians and Gynecologists' Committee on Practice
    Bulletins—Obstetrics. Practice bulletin No. 171: management of preterm labor.
    Obstet Gynecol 2016;128(4):e155–64.
82. Vogel JP, Oladapo OT, Manu A, et al. New WHO recommendations to improve the
    outcomes of preterm birth. Lancet Glob Health 2015;3(10):e589–90.
83. Gentle SJ, Carlo WA, Tan S, et al. Association of antenatal corticosteroids and
    magnesium sulfate therapy with neurodevelopmental outcome in extremely pre-
    term children. Obstet Gynecol 2020;135(6):1377–86.
84. McPheeters ML, Miller WC, Hartmann KE, et al. The epidemiology of threatened
    preterm labor: a prospective cohort study. Am J Obstet Gynecol 2005;192(4):
    1325–9.
85. Brown K, Raghuraman N, Ghartey J, et al. 347: neonatal outcomes in sponta-
    neous versus indicated late preterm birth. Am J Obstet Gynecol 2020;222:
    S232–3.
86. Tuppurainen N, Hallman M. Prevention of neonatal group B streptococcal dis-
    ease: intrapartum detection and chemoprophylaxis of heavily colonized parturi-
    ents. Obstet Gynecol 1989;73(4):583–7.
87. Roberts D, Dalziel S. Antenatal corticosteroids for accelerating fetal lung matura-
    tion for women at risk of preterm birth. Cochrane Database Syst Rev
    2006;(3):CD004454.
88. Brownfoot FC, Gagliardi DI, Bain E, et al. Different corticosteroids and regimens
    for accelerating fetal lung maturation for women at risk of preterm birth. Cochrane
    Database Syst Rev 2013;(8):CD006764.
89. Mercer BM, Miodovnik M, Thurnau GR, et al. Antibiotic therapy for reduction of
    infant morbidity after preterm premature rupture of the membranes: a random-
    ized controlled trial. JAMA 1997;278(12):989–95.
90. Mercer BM, Rabello YA, Thurnau GR, et al. The NICHD-MFMU antibiotic treat-
    ment of preterm PROM study: impact of initial amniotic fluid volume on pregnancy
    outcome. Am J Obstet Gynecol 2006;194(2):438–45.
91. Flenady V, Wojcieszek AM, Papatsonis DN, et al. Calcium channel blockers for
    inhibiting preterm labour and birth. Cochrane Database Syst Rev
    2014;(6):CD002255.
92. Reinebrant HE, Pileggi-Castro C, Romero CL, et al. Cyclo-oxygenase (COX) in-
    hibitors for treating preterm labour. Cochrane Database Syst Rev
    2015;(6):CD001992.

Current Preterm Birth Prevention Strategies

Noelle Breslin, MD[a], Cynthia Gyamfi-Bannerman, MD, MSc[b],*

KEYWORDS

- Preterm birth • Cervical length • Cerclage • Progesterone • Pessary

KEY POINTS

- Preterm birth is a significant source of neonatal and childhood morbidity and mortality worldwide.
- Identifying those at risk of preterm birth, based on obstetric and gynecologic history, demographics, previous preterm birth, and cervical length screening allows for timely intervention in order to attempt to reduce the rates of preterm birth.
- Universal cervical length screening may aid in identifying both those women considered low as well as high-risk women at risk of preterm birth.

INTRODUCTION

Preterm birth is the leading cause of neonatal and childhood mortality under the age of 5 years worldwide.[1–4] An inverse relationship exists between gestational age at delivery and risks of neonatal morbidity and mortality.[5,6] In those children who survive, prematurity secondary to preterm birth is a significant cause of morbidity, prolonged hospitalizations, and long-term health consequences, which affects families and society at large. The Institute of Medicine estimated the cost of preterm birth (PTB) treatment, including neonatal interventions, care for up to 5 years, and disability-specific costs including loss of productivity income, to be $26 billion dollars annually in the United States.[7] However, the actual cost is likely to extend beyond financial expenses and include emotional and psychosocial consequences such as postpartum depression and anxiety, which are more likely to occur in women who deliver preterm.[8]

The incidence of preterm birth varies between countries with the global incidence of preterm birth cited as 10.6% of live births or 14.8 million preterm births.[9] These figures are marred by gaps in data, poor-quality data, and differences in reporting systems. This most often occurs in low-income countries where pregnancy dating by ultrasound is not available and unreliable methods such as last menstrual period estimation,

[a] Columbia University Irving Medical Center, Department of Maternal and Fetal Medicine, 622 West 168th Street, Ph 12-28, New York, NY 10032, USA; [b] Maternal-Fetal Medicine Fellowship Program, Columbia University, CUMC Preterm Birth Prevention Center, 630 West 168th Street, PH-16, New York, NY 10032, USA
* Corresponding author.
E-mail address: cg2231@cumc.columbia.edu

Clin Perinatol 47 (2020) 705–717
https://doi.org/10.1016/j.clp.2020.08.001
0095-5108/20/© 2020 Elsevier Inc. All rights reserved.
perinatology.theclinics.com

fundal height, and birth weight are used as a proxy for pregnancy dating. Further, gestational age definitions of preterm delivery vary, such that, the true incidence of preterm birth on a global scale remains uncertain.[10]

PTB can be categorized as spontaneous or indicated. Spontaneous preterm birth occurs in women who present with labor complaints or premature rupture of membranes. Indicated preterm birth is initiated by the obstetrician in the absence of spontaneous labor due to pregnancy-related maternal complications such as preeclampsia, eclampsia, worsening organ dysfunction, and vaginal bleeding with maternal instability or for fetal indications such as nonreassuring fetal testing. Both these categories of preterm birth are targets of intervention and research to decrease their occurrence.

Although very early preterm birth (<28 weeks of gestation) is associated with the highest neonatal morbidity and mortality, most preterm births occur in the late preterm period (34 + 0–36 + 6 weeks gestation).[11] Although these deliveries occur near term, they are still associated with greater morbidity and greater health care needs than those born at term. The recognition of this preterm birth—associated morbidity led the obstetric community to make a concerted effort to reduce nonmedically indicated preterm birth.[12] In the United States, preterm birth, defined as less than 37 weeks of gestation at delivery, accounted for 10.2% of live births in 2018. This figure has decreased from a peak of 12.8% in 2006.[13,14] A population-based retrospective analysis of PTB data in the United States found a decline in spontaneous PTB by 15.4% and indicated preterm birth by 17.2% between 2005 and 2012. The decline in the overall rate of PTB in the United States is due in part to a reduction in later PTB with a 15.8% reduction in late preterm birth reported over this time period.[13] Although rates have been declining, PTB still remains a significant cause of neonatal morbidity and mortality especially in low-income regions. Identification of PTB risk factors to allow intervention and prevention strategies remain an important goal of researchers in order to reduce the significant burden of preterm birth.

RISK FACTORS FOR RECURRENT PRETERM BIRTH

In order to identify areas of PTB intervention and prevention, we need to understand the risk factors for PTB (**Table 1**). Maternal ethnicity, age, smoking history, periodontal disease, body mass index (BMI), and socioeconomic status are all associated with adverse pregnancy outcomes including a risk of preterm birth. Although race and ethnicity are unmodifiable risk factors, the recognition of racial disparities in terms of preterm birth risk is important in helping to identify those women who require assistance with access to care, patient education, and cervical length screening. Teen pregnancy, short interval pregnancy, BMI, and smoking are modifiable risk factors that are amenable to preconceptual counseling, patient education, and early intervention strategies.

Table 1
Risk factors for preterm birth

Modifiable	Nonmodifiable
• Age	• Race
• Smoking	• Ethnicity
• Obesity	
• Socioeconomic status	
• Periodontal disease	
• Short interval pregnancy	

One of the strongest predictors of PTB is previous PTB with a 1.5- to 2-fold increase risk of PTB in a subsequent pregnancy with the number of previous PTB and gestational age at delivery strongly influencing recurrence.[15]

SCREENING FOR PRETERM BIRTH PREVENTION
Cervical Length Screening

Cervical length, best measured by transvaginal ultrasound is a cost-effective, safe, and acceptable method to identify women at risk of preterm birth, as we know the risk of spontaneous preterm birth is increased in women with a midpregnancy short cervix.[16–18] Once the cervical length reduces to less than or equal to 25 mm, the risk of PTB will have more than doubled.[17] The recognition of a short cervix allows for interventions such as progesterone supplementation for those without a prior preterm birth or cerclage in those with a history of preterm birth. Despite these findings, the utility of universal cervical length screening in low-risk women, that is, those without a history of preterm birth, is still being debated in the medical literature. Proponents for universal screen cite the practice as low cost and low risk with the potential for identifying those who would benefit from intervention to reduce PTB, whereas opponents cite concern regarding lack of quality assessment, poor access for certain populations, and the risk of overtreatment for women who may never have proceeded to have a PTB. The American College of Obstetricians and Gynecologists (ACOG) does not mandate universal cervical length screening but recognizes that it may be considered for low-risk women.[18] The society for maternal and fetal medicine (SMFM) state that screening in singleton gestations without prior preterm birth cannot be universally mandated yet but is considered "reasonable" and may be considered by individual providers. Should providers decide to implement universal screening, strict guidelines for screening should be used.[19]

Other screening methods including screening for bacterial vaginosis, asymptomatic bacteriuria, or uterine activity monitoring have not been proved to improve perinatal outcomes and are currently not recommended as standard.

CURRENT PREVENTION STRATEGIES
Progesterone Supplementation

Supplemental progesterone has been found to be protective against preterm birth in a subset of women. The exact mechanism of action remains unclear. It is known that cervical remodeling is necessary to allow for dilation and delivery. Progesterone withdrawal occurs before delivery during the cervical ripening phase so that supplementation may prevent preterm cervical remodeling.[20] However, the true role of progesterone in cervical remodeling remains uncertain.

17-alpha hydroxyprogesterone caproate
Women with a previous preterm delivery are known to be at high risk of recurrence, and intramuscular progesterone has been used to prevent preterm birth in this setting. In 2003, Meis and colleagues reported a 34% reduction in the rate of PTB less than 37 weeks' gestation in women with a prior PTB when intramuscular progesterone was administered in a double-blind randomized controlled trial. There were 310 women in the progesterone group and the 153 women in the placebo group. The investigators found that treatment with 17P significantly reduced the risk of delivery at less than 37 weeks of gestation by 37%, and the trial was halted early due to the detection of significance of outcome.[21] Fonseca and colleagues, also reported a reduction in PTB in women at high risk of PTB with progesterone supplementation via the vaginal route in a double-blind randomized controlled trial involving 142

high-risk singleton pregnancies. Vaginal progesterone was associated with a significant reduction in preterm birth compared with placebo.[22]

Although initially, society recommendations endorsed treatment of women with a prior PTB with progesterone in either formulation, further studies suggested a preferential benefit of 17-hydroxyprogesteron (17-OHP) over vaginal progesterone in women with a prior PTB, thus intramuscular progesterone was recommended for prevention of preterm birth in women with a history of spontaneous preterm birth before 37 weeks. The medication was approved by an accelerated pathway by the US Food and Drug Administration (FDA).[23]

In 2020, the results of the PROLONG trial were published in the American Journal of Perinatology, which cast doubt on the recommendations for intramuscular progesterone for the prevention of preterm birth.[24,25] The PROLONG trial was performed as a follow-up to the MEIS trial in order to confirm the findings regarding the utility of intramuscular progesterone for the prevention of spontaneous preterm birth. This confirmatory trial was also required by the FDA in order to continue approval. As such, the FDA was involved in consultation of trial design to ensure it was consistent with the study protocol from the National Institute of Child Health and Human Development (NICHD) Maternal-Fetal Medicine Units (MFMU) trial. The PROLONG trial was a multicenter, randomized, controlled, parallel group, double-blind trial at 93 total centers across 9 countries, with most of the enrolled participants coming from outside of the United States.

The results were unexpected in that the PROLONG study had an almost 50% lower rate of preterm birth than expected and was unable to confirm treatment efficacy. This prompted debate among the obstetric community regarding the use of this medication without proven benefit. Some argue the medication is expensive and painful for women to receive without the proven benefit of a reduction in preterm birth, whereas others note that the trial had very dissimilar populations with a large proportion of women being recruited outside of the United States and a low number of these women with a history of multiple spontaneous preterm births or short cervix. Those with higher risk of recurrent preterm birth may have been less likely to participate given the already wide spread use of 17-alpha hydroxyprogesterone caproate (17-OHPC).

Subsequent guidelines from ACOG state, "Consideration for offering 17-OHPC to women at risk of recurrent preterm birth should continue to consider the body of evidence for progesterone supplementation, the values and preferences of the pregnant woman, the resources available, and the setting in which the intervention will be implemented. Additional information from planned meta-analysis and secondary analyses will need to be evaluated to assess the impact this intervention has on women at risk of recurrent preterm birth in the United States. ACOG is not changing our clinical recommendations at this time."[24]

SMFM released a statement recommending obstetric care providers "use an individualized approach as they council patients regarding the use of 17-OHPC. It is reasonable for providers to continue to use 17-OHPC in the context of a shared decision-making model that includes consideration of risk level for recurrent PTB. Important factors to discuss include: uncertainty regarding the benefit, the lack of short-term safety concerns, the possibility of injection site pain, extra patient visits, and substantial costs." They further recommended additional research on 17-OHPC to identify populations in whom it is likely to be effective.[25]

Vaginal Progesterone

A systematic review and meta-analysis of randomized controlled trials comparing vaginal progesterone with placebo in women with a singleton pregnancy and a short cervix before 24 weeks published in 2012 reported that the use of vaginal progesterone in these cases was associated with a significant reduction in the risk of PTB occurring less than 28 weeks' gestation through to 35 weeks as well as a reduction in adverse neonatal outcomes.[26] Despite some dispute over its effectiveness in the literature,[27] vaginal progesterone has consistently been shown to reduce the risk of PTB in women with a short cervix and no prior history of PTB and represents a safe, acceptable, and cost-effective method to reduce PTB.[28]

Thus, vaginal progesterone is recommended for women with a short cervix and no prior history of preterm birth.

CERVICAL CERCLAGE

A cervical cerclage is a method of surgical management of cervical in sufficiency with the aim to prevent preterm birth. It was first introduced by Shirodkar in 1955[29] in which a circular incision is made in the cervix at the level of the internal cervical os with dissection of the bladder to allow placement of a suture that encircles the cervix. This technique was further simplified by McDonald in 1957 in which a purse string suture is placed in the cervix at the highest possible level without requiring dissection of the bladder.[30]

ACOG provides clear guidelines on indications for cervical cerclage placement in singleton pregnancies and divides these indications into 3 categories (**Table 2**).

History Indicated

A history-indicated cerclage includes those women who have had *one or more* previous second trimester losses. These losses must occur in the setting of painless dilation and in the absence of placental abruption. Alternatively, a cerclage is indicated in a woman with a history of a previous cerclage placement due to painless dilation in the second trimester.

Ultrasound Indicated

A cerclage is indicated in the presence of a short cervix less than 25 mm detected at less than 24 weeks *and* a history of a prior singleton preterm birth at less than

Table 2
Indications and contraindications to cervical cerclage placement

History Indicated	Ultrasound Indicated	Examination Indicated
• One or more second trimester pregnancy losses in relation to painless cervical dilation • Prior examination indicated cerclage placement	• Short cervix (<25 mm) diagnosed on ultrasound before 24 wk gestation in a singleton pregnancy with a history of a prior singleton preterm birth <34 wk gestation	• Painless cervical dilation in the second trimester
Contraindications to Cerclage Placement:		
• A history of preterm birth secondary to abruption or preterm labor	• Short cervix in the absence of previous singleton preterm birth • Short cervix diagnosed in a multiple gestation	• Evidence of preterm premature rupture of membranes • Evidence of abruption • Evidence of labor • Chorioamnionitis

34 weeks. If a woman is diagnosed with an asymptomatic short cervix less than 20 mm before 24 weeks and has no history of preterm birth, vaginal progesterone is indicated.

Physical Examination Indicated

Women who present with cervical dilation in the second trimester less than 24 weeks are candidates for a physical examination–indicated cerclage, in the absence of labor or concern for placental abruption.

Contraindications to Cerclage

Women should not be considered candidates for cervical cerclage in the case of a short cervix (<25 mm) at less than 24 weeks in a woman *without* a history of singleton preterm birth. Similarly, for women with a cervical length less than 25 mm and a twin or higher order multiple pregnancy, cerclage is not currently recommended. There is also a lack of evidence to recommend cerclage in those with prior cervical surgery such as large loop electrosurgical excision, cone biopsy, or Mullerian anomaly (see **Table 2**).

MANAGEMENT OF A TRANSVAGINAL CERCLAGE

After placement of a cerclage for any of the abovementioned indications, further investigation with cervical length surveillance is not recommended.[19]

Transvaginal cerclage removal is recommended to occur at 36 to 37 weeks, in uncomplicated cases. According to ACOG, the purpose of removing a cerclage before the onset of spontaneous labor is to prevent cervical injury if labor and cervical dilation was to occur. There is no evidence that removal of cerclage triggers labor in these patients, and usually cerclage removal can be safely performed in the office. When removing, it is imperative to cut the suture on one side, below the level of the knot, to prevent the suture remaining embedded in the cervical stroma.

In the case of preterm labor complaints, if the patient demonstrates cervical change or progressive vaginal bleeding, as well as symptoms consistent with preterm labor, the cerclage should be removed.

In the case of PPROM, guidance regarding cerclage management is unclear but there is evidence that retention of cerclage, in the absence of signs or symptoms of labor or abruption, is associated with pregnancy prolongation.[31] Regardless, women who PPROM with a cerclage in situ, should be treated in the same manner as a patient without a cerclage in situ with PPROM.

PESSARY

The use of a pessary to prevent preterm birth has been cited since the 1950s using a Bakelite ring to support the structure of the cervix in order to prevent recurrent miscarriage and preterm birth.[32] A pessary, in its various forms, have long been used in gynecology in order to support prolapse of pelvic organs. Their use in obstetrics rests on a similar principle, one of mechanical support for the cervix. A silicone pessary is placed at the cervical os to provide support and allow for redirection of the cervix toward the sacrum, thus changing the mechanical forces on the cervix caused by the growing fetus with the goal being to prevent cervical shortening and preterm birth. However, data on their efficacy Is conflicting, with some small randomized controlled trials showing benefit[33] and others showing no significant difference in the rates of preterm birth.[34] Recent systematic review and meta-analysis also cast doubt on the benefit of the use of pessary to prevent preterm birth for singleton or twin gestations.[35–37] The benefit of pessary for prevention of preterm birth continues to be investigated. An MFMU Network's randomized trial of pessary in singleton pregnancies with a short cervix, funded by the NICHD, in which an Arabin pessary is used in singleton pregnancies with a cervical length less than 20 mm, is eagerly awaited.[36] Similarly, the PROSPECT trial is an MFMU evaluating the use of micronized vaginal progesterone or pessary versus control (placebo) to prevent early preterm birth in women carrying twins and with a cervical length of less than 30 mm[38]

TOCOLYTICS

As contractions are the most common symptom and sign of impending preterm birth, tocolytic medications aim to prevent or reduce the efficacy or frequency of uterine contractions. The ultimate goal of the use of tocolytic medications is to allow the administration of steroids for fetal lung maturity, allow administration of magnesium for fetal neuroprotection, and/or allow for maternal transport to a facility skilled in the management of preterm neonates. Tocolytic medications are not without adverse maternal or possible fetal adverse effects, thus they are recommended for short-term use to allow for administration of antenatal corticosteroids only and are not recommended for prolonged usage.[39] The most commonly used agents include nonsteroidal antiinflammatory drugs and calcium channel blockers. Indomethacin is not used beyond 32 weeks of gestation due to concern regarding premature constriction of the ductus arteriosus with administration in the late third trimester. Contraindications to tocolysis include the presence of an intrauterine demise or lethal anomaly where prolonging maturity would be of no benefit. Nonreassuring fetal status, chorioamnionitis, maternal bleeding with hemodynamic instability, or severe maternal conditions such as severe preeclampsia or eclampsia are also contraindications (**Table 3**), as prolonging gestation is likely to lead to harmful fetal and maternal effects. The use of tocolytics in the setting of preterm premature rupture of membranes is controversial but they may be considered in the absence of maternal infection for the purposes of allowing for steroid administration and/or maternal transport.[39]

PREVENTION STRATEGIES FOR MULTIPLE GESTATIONS

Women with multiple gestations are six times more likely to give birth preterm and up to thirteen times more likely to give birth before 32 weeks.[40] Cervical length screening can help identify those women at risk of preterm birth; however, multiple gestations represent a particularly challenging group when it comes to preterm birth prevention and Indicates that the cause of preterm birth among multiple gestations differs to that of singletons, this likely explains the fact that interventions found to be useful in singletons in preventing recurrent preterm birth have not been consistently

Table 3
Contraindications to tocolysis
• Lethal fetal anomaly
• Intrauterine fetal demise
• Nonreassuring fetal status
• Chorioamnionitis
• Preterm premature rupture of membranes*
• Maternal bleeding with hemodynamic instability
• Maternal contraindications to tocolysis medication
• Severe preeclampsia or ecl
• Tocolytics may be considered in PPROM in order to allow for transport or steroid administration in the absence of additional contraindications to tocolysis

proved to be beneficial in multiple gestations. Although cerclage has been proved to be beneficial in singleton pregnancies, ACOG recommends against the placement of cervical cerclages in multiple gestations,[40] as previous studies have not shown benefit in preventing preterm birth in women without a history of cervical insufficiency or in those with a short cervix.[41] Similarly, prophylactic tocolytics are not recommended in multiple gestations.[40] The use of a pessary in the prevention of preterm birth for multiple gestations has also not been proved to be beneficial in multiple gestations and at present is not recommended for use in multiple gestations.[42] In addition, the use of supplementary progesterone has not been shown to be beneficial for use in multiple gestations.[43–46] This leaves little in the arsenal of the obstetrician in preventing preterm birth in twins and higher order multiple gestations. Research into the prevention of preterm birth in twins and higher order multiples is ongoing.

REDUCING IATROGENIC PRETERM BIRTH

Iatrogenic or indicated PTB occurs in the setting of fetal or maternal indications for delivery with the aim of decreasing maternal and/or fetal morbidity or mortality. In order to reduce iatrogenic preterm birth, we must look at the factors that contribute to iatrogenic preterm birth and develop strategies for prevention.

In Vitro Fertilization Practices

As mentioned previously, multiple gestations have an increased incidence of preterm birth. With the increased use of in vitro fertilization (IVF) and fertility treatments, a concerted effort in reducing the incidence of multiple gestations has been made with the American Society of Reproductive Medicine (ASRM) providing guidelines to the number of embryos to be transferred with a single embryo transfer preferred for women with euploid embryos regardless of maternal age.[47] Similarly, for women who require ovulation induction with gonadotrophins, ASRM recommends close monitoring of the treatment cycle and use of a low-dose treatment with cautious medication titration as needed to attain monofollicular development.[48]

Multifetal Pregnancy Reduction

Higher order multiple gestations are associated with high rates of not only spontaneous PTB but also iatrogenic PTB due to the increased risks of maternal morbidity, fetal growth complications, and in some cases, the intrinsic complications associated with a shared placental circulation in monochorionic pairs. Should a higher order multiple gestation occur, either spontaneously or via fertility treatment, consideration for selective reduction of a multiple pregnancy should be discussed with the patient. Multifetal pregnancy reduction (MFPR) is the process of reducing a higher order multiple gestation to twins or a singleton pregnancy in order to reduce the fetal as well as maternal perinatal morbidity and mortality associated with higher order multiple gestations. MFPR has been shown to improve the preterm birth rate in triplet pregnancies by approximately 1 month and neonatal weight by approximately 1 pound. In addition, both neonatal morbidity and mortality are reduced with improved long-term neurocognitive outcomes.[49] Reduction of triplets to singleton has been shown to result in improved obstetric outcomes when compared with reduction to twins, without increasing procedure-related complications.[50] However, the decision as to how many fetuses to reduce is a deeply personal and should be made after detailed patient counseling by a maternal fetal medicine physician who can explain the risks and benefits of all available options. Detailed ultrasound should be performed to determine chorionicity and to assess for obvious structural anomalies, which may guide which fetus to reduce. Genetic analysis is strongly recommended. Because the procedure is carried out between 11 to 13 weeks, chorionic villus sampling before the procedure is recommended to ensure the remaining fetus or fetuses are euploid. The procedure is recommended to occur in a specialized fetal therapy center.

Selective Termination

Selective termination is the term used to describe a targeted reduction of one or more fetuses due to a diagnosis of a structural, genetic, or growth abnormality. It may also be indicated in cases of monochorionic twin gestation complicated by twin to twin transfusion syndrome where fetoscopic laser ablation is either not desirable or unattainable to the patient. The goal with selective termination is to optimize outcomes for the remaining fetus/fetuses by reducing the risk of iatrogenic preterm birth indicated by either fetal testing, maternal well-being, or both.

Aspirin

Iatrogenic preterm birth is not only guided by fetal well-being but is also driven by maternal well-being. Maternal hypertensive disease, including worsening chronic hypertension, preeclampsia, or eclampsia are all drivers for delivery. Aspirin has been shown to reduce the risk of preeclampsia in women with factors considered high risk for the development of preeclampsia when administered daily after initiated between 12 and 28 weeks of gestation and continued until delivery.[51] The indications for aspirin therapy for preeclampsia prophylaxis are demonstrated in **Table 4**.

Table 4 Recommendations for Aspirin use to prevent preeclampsia	
High-Risk Factors	**Recommend Aspirin Use**
• History of preeclampsia, especially if associated with an adverse outcome • Chronic hypertension • Multiple gestation • Pregestational diabetes • Renal disease • Autoimmune disease	One or more high-risk factors
Moderate Risk Factors	**Consider Aspirin Use**
• Nulliparity • Age 35 y or older • Obesity • History of preeclampsia i n mother or sister • Sociodemographic factors (low socioeconomic status, African American) • Personal history factors: >10-y pregnancy interval, prior adverse pregnancy outcome, low birth weight or small for gestational age	Two or more moderate-risk factors
Low risk factor: • Previous uncomplicated full-term delivery	**Do Not Recommend Aspirin Use**

In 2020, Hoffman and colleagues published the findings of the Aspirin Supplementation for Pregnancy Indicated Risk Reduction in Nulliparas study. This was a multi-country, double-blind, placebo controlled trial in singleton, nulliparous gestations. The investigators found that the administration of aspirin was associated with a decreased incidence of preterm birth, very preterm birth, and perinatal mortality.[52,53]

Statins

Preeclampsia is a frequent indicator for iatrogenic PTB and is known to have a similar pathogenesis and risk factors to cardiovascular disease. Statins, a class of drug that inhibits the 3-hydroxy-3-methylglutaryl-coenzyme A reductase enzyme, have been shown to restore the pathogenic changes seen in preeclampsia in animal models.[54] The use of statins in prevention of preeclampsia is currently under investigation in a randomized controlled clinical trial.[55]

FUTURE DIRECTIONS

As we understand more about the pathophysiological processes behind preterm birth, we are likely to determine targeted areas of intervention. Research into the biomechanics of the cervix may provide valuable insights into novel targets for intervention.

SUMMARY

Preterm birth remains a clinical challenge for obstetricians and neonatologists. Intervention before pregnancy and in early pregnancy may help reduce the risk of spontaneous preterm birth via accessible birth control for teenage girls, monitored ovulation cycles, single embryo transfers, multifetal pregnancy reduction, cerclage placement, progesterone supplementation, and medication for preeclampsia prevention. Optimal strategies for prevention of preterm birth in multiple gestations remains to be elucidated. PTB will likely remain a significant issue for perinatologists; identification and counseling of women at risk of preterm birth is important in allowing women to understands the risks of these complications in pregnancy and neonatal life.

REFERENCES

1. Goldenberg RL, Culhane JF, Iams JD, et al. Epidemiology and causes of preterm birth. Lancet 2008;371(9606):75–84.
2. Manuck IA. Pharmacogenomics of preterm birth prevention and treatment. BJOG 2016;123(3):368–75.
3. Russell RB, Green NS, Steiner CA, et al. Cost of hospitalization for preterm and low birth weight infants in the United States. Pediatrics 2007;120(1):e1–9.
4. Ananth CV, Friedman AM, Gyamfi-Bannerman C. Epidemiology of moderate preterm, late preterm and early term delivery. Clin Perinatol 2013;40(4):601–10.
5. Stoll BJ, Hansen NI, Bell EF, et al. Neonatal outcomes of extremely preterm infants from the NICHD Neonatal research network. Pediatrics 2010;126(3):443–56.
6. Matthews TJ, MacDorman MF, Thoma ME. Infant mortality statistics from the 2013 period linked birth/infant death data set. Natl Vital Stat Rep 2015;64(9):1–30.
7. Behrman RE, Butler AS, editors. Preterm birth: causes, consequences, and prevention. Washington, DC: National Academies Press; 2007.
8. Frey HA, Klebanoff MA. The epidemiology, etiology, and costs of preterm birth. Semin Fetal Neonatal Med 2016;21(2):68–73.
9. Nour NM. Premature delivery and the millennium development goal. Rev Obstet Gynecol 2012;5(2):100–5.

10. Lee AC, Blencowe H, Lawn JE. Small babies, big numbers: global estimates of preterm birth. Lancet Glob Health 2019;7(1):e2–3.

11. Martin JA, Hamilton BE, Osterman MJ, et al. Births: final data for 2013. Natl Vital Stat Rep 2015;64(1):1–65.

12. Gynecologists ACoOa. ACOG committee opinion no. 561: nonmedically indicated early-term deliveries. Obstet Gynecol 2013;121(4):911–5.

13. Gyamfi-Bannerman C, Ananth CV. Trends in spontaneous and indicated preterm delivery among singleton gestations in the United States, 2005-2012. Obstet Gynecol 2014;124(6):1069–74.

14. Centers for disease control and Prevention. National center for health statistics. Available at: https://www.cdc.gov/nchs/nvss/births.htm?CDC_AA_refVal=https%3A%2F%2Fwww.cdc.gov%2Fnchs%2Fbirths.htm. Accessed October 19, 2019).

15. McManemy J, Cooke E, Amon E, et al. Recurrence risk for preterm delivery. Am J Obstet Gynecol 2007;196(6):576.e1-6 [discussion: e6–7].

16. Berghella V, Bega G, Tolosa JE, et al. Ultrasound assessment of the cervix. Clin Obstet Gynecol 2003;46(4):947–62.

17. Iams JD, Goldenberg RL, Meis PJ, et al. The length of the cervix and the risk of spontaneous premature delivery. National institute of child health and human development maternal fetal medicine unit network. N Engl J Med 1996;334(9):567–72.

18. Iams JD, Goldenberg RL, Mercer BM, et al. The preterm prediction study: recurrence risk of spontaneous preterm birth. National institute of child health and human development maternal-fetal medicine units network. Am J Obstet Gynecol 1998;178(5):1035–40.

19. Society for Maternal-Fetal Medicine (SMFM) Publications Committee, McIntosh J, Feltovich H, Berghella V, et al. The role of routine cervical length screening in selected high- and low-risk women for preterm birth prevention. Am J Obstet Gynecol 2016;215(3):B2–7.

20. Vink J, Feltovich H. Cervical etiology of spontaneous preterm birth. Semin Fetal Neonatal Med 2016;21:106–12.

21. Meis PJ, Klebanoff M, Thom E, et al. Prevention of recurrent preterm delivery by 17 alpha-hydroxyprogesterone caproate. N Engl J Med 2003;348(24):2379–85.

22. da Fonseca EB, Bittar RE, Carvalho MH, et al. Prophylactic administration of progesterone by vaginal suppository to reduce the incidence of spontaneous preterm birth in women at increased risk: a randomized placebo-controlled double-blind study. Am J Obstet Gynecol 2003;188(2):419–24.

23. Society for Maternal-Fetal Medicine Publications Committee, with assistance of Vincenzo Berghella. Progesterone and preterm birth prevention: translating clinical trials data into clinical practice. Am J Obstet Gynecol 2012;206(5):376–86.

24. ACOG Practice Advisory: Clinical guidance for integration of the findings of the PROLONG study: progestin's role in optimizing neonatal gestation, ACOG, october 25. Available at: https://www.acog.org/clinical/clinical-guidance/practice-advisory/articles/2019/10/clinical-guidance-for-integration-of-the-findings-of-the-prolong-study. Last accessed 5/6/20).

25. Society for Maternal-Fetal Medicine (SMFM) Publications Committee. SMFM Statement: use of 17-alpha hydroxyprogesterone caproate for prevention of recurrent preterm birth. Am J Obstet Gynecol 2020;223(1):B16–8.

26. Romero R, Nicolaides K, Conde-Agudelo A, et al. Vaginal progesterone in women with an asymptomatic sonographic short cervix in the midtrimester decreases

preterm delivery and neonatal morbidity: a systematic review and metaanalysis of individual patient data. Am J Obstet Gynecol 2012;206(2):124.e1-19.

27. Norman JE, Marlow N, Messow CM, et al. Vaginal progesterone prophylaxis for preterm birth (the OPPTIMUM study): a multicentre, randomised, double-blind trial. Lancet 2016;387(10033):2106–16.

28. Romero R, Conde-Agudelo A, Da Fonseca E, et al. Vaginal progesterone for preventing preterm birth and adverse perinatal outcomes in singleton gestations with a short cervix: a meta-analysis of individual patient data. Am J Obstet Gynecol 2018;218(2):161–80.

29. Shirodkar VN. A new method of operative treatment for habitual abortion in the second trimester of pregnancy. Antiseptic 1955;52:299.

30. Simcox R, Shennan A. Cervical cerclage: a review. Int J Surg 2007;5(3):205–9.

31. Giraldo-Isaza MA, Berghella V. Cervical cerclage and preterm PROM. Clin Obstet Gynecol 2011;54(2):313–20.

32. Cross RG. Treatment of habitual abortion due to cervical incompetence. Lancet 1959;2:127.

33. Goya M, Pratcorona L, Merced C, et al. Cervical pessary in pregnant women with a short cervix (PECEP): an open-label randomised controlled trial. Lancet 2012; 379(9828):1800–6.

34. Nicolaides KH, Syngelaki A, Poon LC, et al. Cervical pessary placement for prevention of preterm birth in unselected twin pregnancies: a randomized controlled trial. Am J Obstet Gynecol 2016;214(1):3.e1–9.

35. Conde-Agudelo A, Romero R, Nicolaides KH. Cervical pessary to prevent preterm birth in asymptomatic high-risk women: a systematic review and meta-analysis. Am J Obstet Gynecol 2020;223(1):42–65.e2.

36. Jarde A, Lutsiv O, Beyene J, et al. Vaginal progesterone, oral progesterone, 17-OHPC, cerclage, and pessary for preventing preterm birth in at-risk singleton pregnancies: an updated systematic review and network meta-analysis. BJOG 2019;126(5):556–67.

37. ClinicalTrials.gov. A randomized trial of pessary in singleton pregnancies with a short cervix (TOPS). Available at: https://clinicaltrials.gov/ct2/show/NCT02901626 (Last accessed 4/24/20).

38. ClinicalTrials.gov. A trial of pessary and progesterone and preterm prevention in twin gestation with a short cervix (PROSPECT). Available at: https://clinicaltrials.gov/ct2/show/NCT02518594 (Last accessed 7/26/20).

39. American College of Obstetricians and Gynecologists, Committee on Practice Bulletins—Obstetrics. ACOG practice bulletin no. 127: management of preterm labor. Obstet Gynecol 2012;119(6):1308–17.

40. American College of Obstetricians and Gynecologists, Society for Maternal-Fetal Medicine. ACOG practice bulletin no. 144: multifetal gestations: twin, triplet, and higher-order multifetal pregnancies. Obstet Gynecol 2014;123(5):1118–32.

41. Rafael TJ, Berghella V, Alfirevic Z. Cervical stitch (cerclage) for preventing preterm birth in multiple pregnancy. Cochrane Database Syst Rev 2014;9: CD009166.

42. Liem S, Schuit E, Hegeman M, et al. Cervical pessaries for prevention of preterm birth in women with a multiple pregnancy (ProTWIN): a multicentre, open-label randomised controlled trial. Lancet 2013;382(9901):1341–9.

43. Senat MV, Porcher R, Winer N, et al. Prevention of preterm delivery by 17 alpha-hydroxyprogesterone caproate in asymptomatic twin pregnancies with a short cervix: a randomized controlled trial. Am J Obstet Gynecol 2013;208(3):194.e1-8.

44. Serra V, Perales A, Meseguer J, et al. Increased doses of vaginal progesterone for the prevention of preterm birth in twin pregnancies: a randomised controlled double-blind multicentre trial. BJOG 2013;120(1):50–7.
45. Caritis SN, Rouse DJ, Peaceman AM, et al. Prevention of preterm birth in triplets using 17 alpha-hydroxyprogesterone caproate: a randomized controlled trial. Obstet Gynecol 2009;113(2 Pt 1):285–92.
46. Rouse DJ, Caritis SN, Peaceman AM, et al. A trial of 17 alpha-hydroxyprogesterone caproate to prevent prematurity in twins. N Engl J Med 2007;357(5):454–61.
47. ASRM@asrm.org PCotASfRMEa, Technology PCotSfAR. Guidance on the limits to the number of embryos to transfer: a committee opinion. Fertil Steril 2017;107(4): 901–3.
48. asrm@asrm.org PCotASfRMaSfREalEa. Use of exogenous gonadotropins for ovulation induction in anovulatory women: a committee opinion. Fertil Steril 2020;113(1):66–70.
49. Običan S, Brock C, Berkowitz R, et al. Multifetal pregnancy reduction. Clin Obstet Gynecol 2015;58(3):574–84.
50. Zemet R, Haas J, Bart Y, et al. Pregnancy outcome after multifetal pregnancy reduction of triplets to twins versus reduction to singletons. Reprod Biomed Online 2020;40(3):445–52.
51. Meher S, Duley L, Hunter K, et al. Antiplatelet therapy before or after 16 weeks' gestation for preventing preeclampsia: an individual participant data meta-analysis. Am J Obstet Gynecol 2017;216(2):121–8.e2.
52. Hoffman MK, Goudar SS, Kodkany BS, et al. Low dose aspirin for the prevention of preterm delivery in nulliparous women with a singleton pregnancy (ASPIRIN): a randomized, double-blind, placebo-controlled trial. Lancet 2020;395:285–93.
53. Andrikopoulou M, Purisch SE, Handal-Orefice R, et al. Low dose aspirin is associated with reduced spontaneous preterm birth in nulliparous women. Am J Obstet Gynecol 2018;219:399.e1–6.
54. Fox KA, Longo M, Tamayo E, et al. Effects of pravastatin on mediators of vascular function in a mouse model of soluble Fms-like tyrosine kinase-1-induced preeclampsia. Am J Obstet Gynecol 2011;205(4)::366.e1-5.
55. Clinicaltrials.gov. Pravastatin for prevention of Preeclampsia (statin). Available at: https://clinicaltrials.gov/ct2/show/NCT01717586?term=statins&cond=Preterm+Birth&draw=2&rank=4. Accessed April 28. 2020.

Neurologic Outcomes After Prenatal Treatment of Twin-Twin Transfusion Syndrome

Desmond Sutton, MD, Russell Miller, MD*

KEYWORDS

- Twin-twin transfusion syndrome • Fetoscopic laser surgery • Fetoscopy
- Amnioreduction • Neurologic morbidity • Cerebral palsy

KEY POINTS

- Fetoscopic laser surgery seems to have perinatal survival and neurologic morbidity benefits when compared with amnioreduction for the treatment of early onset, advanced-stage twin-twin transfusion syndrome (TTTS).
- Earlier gestational age at birth, low birthweight, and higher stage of twin-twin transfusion at diagnosis may be associated with poorer neurologic outcomes after laser therapy.
- Although neuroimaging can increase antenatal detection of those pediatric survivors at risk for subsequent neurologic morbidity after laser, full assessment or neurologic status requires pediatric follow-up at 2 years of age or greater.
- The rate of major neurologic morbidity among pediatric survivors of TTTS treated with laser varies from as low as 4% to as high as 18%, with most of the reviews revealing rates less than 10%.

INTRODUCTION

Twin births account for approximately 3% of United States' live births, with roughly 70% of these the result of dizygotic fertilization. Although the prevalence of dizygotic twins varies worldwide among populations, occurrence of the less common monozygotic twins is relatively stable across groups at 3 to 5 per 1000 births.[1,2] Twin pregnancies possess considerable fetal, obstetric, and maternal risks. Perinatal morbidity and mortality are increased, with some reports indicating that fetal death is up to 6 times higher in twins compared with singleton gestations, with observed rates varying based on chorionicity.[3,4] A large proportion of this increased risk derives from higher rates of

Funding source: R.S. Miller disclosed receiving honorarium for writing a article on TRAP sequence for UpToDate. D. Sutton has no disclosures.
Division of Maternal-Fetal Fetal Medicine, Department of Obstetrics and Gynecology, Columbia University College of Physicians and Surgeons, 622 West 168th Street, PH16-66, New York, NY 10032, USA
* Corresponding author.
E-mail address: rsm20@cumc.columbia.edu

Clin Perinatol 47 (2020) 719–731
https://doi.org/10.1016/j.clp.2020.08.002
0095-5108/20/© 2020 Elsevier Inc. All rights reserved.

perinatology.theclinics.com

preterm birth (PTB), preterm rupture of membranes (PPROM), fetal growth restriction, and fetal anomalies in unselected twin pregnancies compared with singleton gestations.

Monochorionic twin gestations present disproportionately higher risk for perinatal morbidity and mortality when compared with their dichorionic twin counterparts due to their potential to develop specific complications attributable to a shared placenta and intertwin placental circulation. A prime example of a monochorionic-specific complication is twin-twin transfusion syndrome (TTTS), a condition affecting 8% to 10% of monochorionic, diamniotic (MCDA) twin gestations in which one twin preferentially shunts blood to its monochorionic co-twin, placing both twins at substantial risk for poor outcomes. Even when excluding monochorionicity-specific disorders such as TTTS from analyses, studies have shown that monochorionic pregnancies remain at higher risk of PTB, small for gestational age birth weight, twin intraventricular hemorrhage (IVH), and neonatal intensive care unit admission.[5]

Established therapies exist for the treatment of TTTS that can reduce risk of perinatal morbidity and mortality, including amnioreduction and fetoscopic laser photocoagulation (laser surgery) of communicating placental anastomoses. Laser surgery has been established as the standard of care for the treatment of early onset, advanced-stage TTTS, offering clear twin survival advantages over amnioreduction and expectant management.[6] The focus of this article is to review the literature regarding neurologic outcomes among pediatric survivors of TTTS.

TWIN-TWIN TRANSFUSION SYNDROME

TTTS is caused by pathologic intertwin anastomoses allowing for unbalanced shunting of blood and vasoactive mediators between twins. It occurs most commonly in MCDA gestations, although all monochorionic multiple gestations are at risk.[7–9] Ultrasound is the mainstay of TTTS diagnosis and evaluation, with a sonographic diagnosis requiring the identification of oligohydramnios in the donor twin and polyhydramnios in the recipient twin. A staging system exists for disease severity that considers twin amniotic fluid volumes, urinary bladder volume status, Doppler velocimetry studies of selected vessels, hydropic changes, and/or fetal death.[10] This system is used to counsel patients regarding prognosis and options, to consider potential candidates for therapy, and to allow for research comparisons.

Although there is currently clinical equipoise regarding the optimal management of stage I disease, it is widely accepted that intervention is recommended for stage II to IV TTTS[8] due to a substantial risk of perinatal morbidity and mortality with untreated early onset advanced-stage TTTS.

AMNIOREDUCTION FOR TWIN-TWIN TRANSFUSION SYNDROME TREATMENT

Amnioreduction involves ultrasound-guided drainage of excess amniotic fluid from the recipient twin's amniotic sac for therapeutic benefit. Before the development of fetoscopic laser surgery, amnioreduction represented first-line treatment of TTTS. The goal of amnioreduction is to reduce uterine distention and thereby lower the risk of preterm labor and PPROM. It can also reduce maternal discomfort. It has additionally been theorized to increase donor twin placental perfusion, although this theory is unproved.[11]

Mari and colleagues[12] described outcomes of 223 sets of twins who were treated with serial aggressive amnioreduction for TTTS from an international TTTS registry of cases from 1990 to 1998. They reported an overall perinatal survival of 78% that dropped to 60% 4 weeks after birth, with 48.4% dual survival and 70.8% survival of at least one twin. Of those neonates who survived to 4 weeks, abnormal findings on cranial (neuroanatomical) imaging were detected in 18%. Intertwin hemoglobin difference at birth was the only one of 19 antenatal and neonatal factors examined to be predictive of abnormal neuroimaging.

FETOSCOPIC LASER SURGERY FOR TWIN-TWIN TRANSFUSION SYNDROME TREATMENT

Laser therapy was first described by De Lia and colleagues[13] in 1990 and involved introduction of a fetoscope with laser fiber into the recipient sac after maternal laparotomy to visualize and photocoagulate placental surface vessels. It has since evolved into a percutaneous fetoscopic technique involving a selective approach for preferentially targeting intertwin anastomoses. Following early single-center experiences suggesting benefit to laser as a treatment of TTTS, the Eurofetus randomized controlled trial (RCT) was conducted. The Eurofetus RCT compared laser with amnioreduction and was concluded early due to proven benefit in favor of laser surgery on interim analysis. In this landmark trial, patients who underwent laser had a higher likelihood of perinatal survival of at least one twin (76% vs 56%, $P = .009$), as well as survival of at least one twin at 6 months of age (76% vs 51%, $P = .002$). Dual twin survivorship at 6 months was higher in the laser group (36% vs 26%) compared with those treated with amnioreduction. In addition, infants had lower rates of cystic periventricular leukomalacia (6% vs 14%, $P = 0.02$) on neuroimaging, with lower reported neurologic morbidity at 6 months (52% vs 31%, $P = .003$).

A smaller multicenter trial comparing laser therapy with amnioreduction was also prematurely discontinued, yet this study did not detect differences in one or both twin survival at 30 days of life.[14] Perhaps as a result of this, a Cochrane meta-analysis in 2014 evaluated 3 trials including 506 fetuses that underwent treatment of TTTS, including 2 that compared amnioreduction with laser. Among these 2 trials, there was no difference in overall death between amnioreduction and laser coagulation or death of at least one or both infants per pregnancy. However, more babies were alive without neurologic abnormality at 6 years in the laser group than in the amnioreduction groups (risk ratio 1.57; 95% confidence interval [CI] 1.05–2.34). This meta-analysis notwithstanding, laser surgery is generally regarded as the superior treatment of the management of advanced-stage TTTS.

As the laser procedure has become more widely available and providers have gained experience, clinical publications have suggested posttrial improvements in survival outcomes. One literature review of more than 2000 cases revealed a perinatal survival of 65%, with 50% of cases having dual survivorship.[7] A systematic review that spanned 25 years of Selective Laser Photocoagulation (SLP) found that survival increased significantly over the time period.[15] As survivorship therefore seems to be improving, the question for survivors becomes "what kind of survival?," and this requires an evaluation of the literature regarding neurologic outcomes after treatment of TTTS.

NEUROLOGIC OUTCOMES AFTER AMNIOREDUCTION FOR TWIN-TWIN TRANSFUSION SYNDROME

Neurologic impairment is a key pediatric outcome measure among survivors, and for some parents it can be more important than overall survival. Compared with singleton pregnancies, unselected twin gestations are at higher risk of neurologic morbidity. Scher and colleagues[16,17] reported on 25,772 twin births in 5 populations in the United States and Australia and found that twins had a 4-fold increase in risk when compared with singletons. Undoubtedly, a significant proportion of this difference is due to the increased prevalence of monochorionicity-associated disorders of pregnancy and PTB among twins.

Scant published data exist describing neurologic outcomes among survivors of expectantly managed advanced-stage TTTS, although major neuromorbidity rates are generally believed to be high. Published neurodevelopmental outcomes after amnioreduction for TTTS are restricted to several series that provide limited data and varied findings. Discrepancies between studies are likely due to differences in methodology, small sample sizes, and heterogeneity within case series. Xiangqun and colleagues examined all pregnancies with TTTS at a single center from 1996 to 2004, in which 62% of cases were treated with amnioreduction. They identified 20 survivors and overall found 30% with neurodevelopmental impairment, including 20% with major neurodevelopmental impairment (cerebral palsy [CP], intelligence quotient <70, deafness, or blindness). Of those with major neurodevelopmental impairment, all received amnioreduction as a treatment 1 to 4 times.[18] Reisner observed an 18% rate of CP among a comparably small cohort of survivors who underwent prenatal amnioreduction.[18] Graef and colleagues[19] collected 6 series (including the Reisner experience) that provided data on neurologic outcomes among 194 amnioreduction survivors. They showed a rate of neurologic abnormality ranging from 7% to 26% for major disability and 11% to 33% for minor. Finally, Van Klink and colleagues reviewed papers that described neurodevelopmental outcomes in survivors of TTTS treated with amnioreduction and reported a 19.9% (range 14%–26%) average rate of impairment, including 13.9% affected with CP (5%–23%).

NEUROLOGIC OUTCOMES AFTER LASER SURGERY FOR TWIN-TWIN TRANSFUSION SYNDROME

There is a range of neurologic outcomes reported in the literature among survivors of laser surgery for TTTS (**Table 1**). A review of more than 1300 pregnancies examined neurodevelopmental outcomes after laser surgery at a median pediatric age of 21 to 26 months and found rates of minor impairment of 7% to 11% and severe impairment (defined as the presence of at least one of the following: CP, severe motor skills delay or cognitive developmental delay, bilateral blindness, or deafness) that ranged from 3% to 11%.[20] In the authors' review, rate of major neurologic morbidity among pediatric survivors of TTTS treated with laser varies from as low as 4% to as high as 18%, with most of the reviews revealing rates less than 10%.

Some literature suggests that neurologic morbidity among twins with TTTS treated with laser and gestational age-matched dichorionic twins may be similar, perhaps suggesting that laser surgery can limit monochorionicity-associated contributions to pediatric neurologic morbidity. Spurijt and colleagues performed a case-control study on cerebral injury detected by postnatal cranial ultrasound. They matched 267 monochorionic twins with TTTS treated with laser with 267 dichorionic twins for gestational age at birth. Incidence of severe cerebral lesions, such as IVH grade III, periventricular hemorrhagic infarction, periventricular leukomalacia grade II or greater, porencephalic cysts, arterial stroke, or ventricular dilatation, was not significantly different between the TTTS and dichorionic twins cohort (8.6% vs 6.7%, P = .44). On multivariate analysis, only gestational age at birth was independently associated with increased risk of severe lesions (odds ratio [OR] 1.35 for each week, P<.01). Of note, 52% of the cerebral lesions in the TTTS cohort were deemed to be antenatal in origin compared with 16.7% in the control group (OR 8.0, P = .02).[21] This study, however, excluded all cases in which there was a fetal demise of one or both twins, which may have influenced findings.

Table 1
Mortality and major neurologic morbidity after fetoseopic laser for twin-twin transfusion syndrome

Study	Subjects	Follow-up Rate (%)	Year Procedure Performed	Pediatric Age at Assessment for Neurologic Outcomes	Mortality (28 d After Birth)		Major Neurologic Morbidity				
					Overall Survival	Dual Survival	Overall	Single Survivor	Double Survivor	Cerebral Palsy
Sutcliffe et al,[49] 2001	67	80	1995–1999	6 mo to 3 y[b]	NR	NR	9%	0%	13.30%	9%
Banek et al,[50,51] 2003	89	100	1995–1997	14–44 mo[b]	61%	42%	11%	21%	8%	NR
Graef et al,[19] 2006	167	98	1997–1999	4–44 mo[b]	68%	54%	6%	13%	4%	NR
Lopriore et al,[51] 2007	115	100	2000–2003	2 y	70%	75%	17%	NR	NR	7%
Lenclen et al,[52] 2009	88	100	2000–2005	2 y	76.7%	NR	4.6%	NR	NR	11%
Lopriore et al,[29] 2009	278	94	2003–2005	2 y	70%	51%	18%	22%	17%	6%
Salomon et al,[53] 2010	73	95	1999–2002	1, 2, 4, and 5 y[c]	76%	36%	12%	NR	NR	8%
Gray et al,[30] 2011	113	97	2002–2006	2 y	79%	NR	12%	0%	14%	4.4%
Graeve et al,[54] 2012	190	75	1995–1999	6 y	64%	NR	9%	20%	6%	NR
Chang et al,[55] 2012	59	96.7	2005–2010	1 y	66%	80%	7%	NR	NR	5%
Vanderbilt et al,[56] 2014	100	49	2007–2010	2 y	NR	NR	4%	NR	NR	3%
McIntosh et al,[57] 2014	50	84	2006–2008	2–6 y[b]	84%	70%	4%	11%	2%	2%
van Klink et al,[58] 2014[a]	318	97	2000–2005 & 2008–2010	2 y	75%	72%	9%	8%	12%	1%
van Klink et al,[39] 2016	216	92	2008–2012	2 y	75%	62%	4%	NR	NR	3%
Spruijt et al,[23] 2019[a]	434	88	2008–2010 & 2011–2014	2 y	78%	NR	4%	NR	NR	2%

Abbreviation: NR, not reported.
[a] Studies reported on 2 cohorts at different time points but given lack of significant differences between them, these outcomes were reported as aggregates.
[b] Patients were evaluated between the listed age ranges.
[c] Patients were evaluated multiple time pcints at ages listed.

As laser surgery has matured as a procedure, some studies have suggested that outcomes have improved. Vohr and colleagues[22] compared 18- to 22-month cognitive scores among 2 cohorts who delivered preterm during 2 separate time periods and found significantly better outcomes as time progressed. However, the investigators notably used 2 different types of tests to assess both cohorts (BSID-II and BSID-III). Spruijt and colleagues[23,24] performed a similar analysis of 2 cohorts of TTTS survivors who underwent SLP from 2008 to 2010 and 2011 to 2014 and found a nonsignificant trend for improved outcomes, with decreasing rates of severe neurodevelopmental impairment over time (6% vs 3%, $P = .189$). They concluded that improvement in outcome of TTTS has reached a plateau, with low birth weight and prenatal cerebral injury serving as risk factors for poor developmental outcome.

Although fetoscopic laser has been associated with improved outcomes compared with amnioreduction, comparisons for neurodevelopmental impairments are more difficult to interpret, as often those with poorer outcomes are less likely to survive to the age of assessment (X). Still, outcomes seem to be superior with fetoscopic laser among those with long-term survival, which has obvious implications for these children and their parents. A systematic review and meta-analysis found a 7-fold higher risk of severe cerebral injury in live-born children treated with amnioreduction compared with fetoscopic laser (OR 7.69, 95% CI 2.78–20.0, $P = .00$), and for those who survived the neonatal period this risk was 3 times higher (OR 3.23, 95% CI 1.45–7.14, $P = .00$).[25]

NEUROLOGIC MORBIDITY COMPARED BETWEEN DONOR AND RECIPIENT TWINS

In TTTS, donor and recipient twins are each at risk, but face different hemodynamic challenges. Given the different pathophysiological conditions that each twin faces, it is hypothesized that donor twins are at risk for ischemic injuries due to cerebral malperfusion, whereas the recipient twins are at risk for ischemia due to polycythemia-associated vascular sludging as well as hemorrhagic events due to hypertensive, hypervolemic overload.[26] The literature seems to indicate that donors and recipients are at equal risk for cerebral injury after laser surgery. A systematic review and meta-analysis of more than 1000 pregnancies that underwent laser surgery for TTTS found that among survivors, neurologic morbidity did not differ between donors and recipients (9% vs 10%, $P = .66$).[27] However, the investigators recommended caution, as none of the studies they included compared donor with recipient as the primary outcome. In addition, of the 14 studies included in their analysis, all but 2 showed a nonsignificant trend toward improved survival in the recipient twin. This postulated that a significant portion of cerebral injuries may actually take place in the first trimester before laser therapy.

NEUROLOGIC MORBIDITY BASED ON QUINTERO STAGE AT DIAGNOSIS

Initial TTTS stating has been shown to be a predictor of outcomes after laser therapy. Advancing Quintero staging and worsening outcomes have been found to be positively correlated not only for immediate outcomes such as perinatal mortality and morbidity but also for long-term neuromorbidity. In the Eurofetus trial, the investigators found that in fetuses undergoing laser and amnioreduction for TTTS, advancing Quintero stage was associated with lower rates of single survival.[28] The same has held true for long-term follow-up. Lopriore and colleagues[29] examined 212 twin pregnancies that underwent laser surgery for TTTS and found that risk factors for neurologic morbidity included advanced Quintero staging at diagnosis with an OR of 3.55 for each increment increase in stage ($P = .04$). Gray and colleagues[30] reported on 113 children examined 2 years after laser therapy for TTTS and found that advancing stage at diagnosis had a strong association with neurodevelopmental disability (OR 13.02, 95% CI 1.92–88.33). In this study, laser therapy was not offered until stage II or greater TTTS was present. Similar associations have been reported in other studies, as well.

NEUROLOGIC MORBIDITY AFTER SINGLE TWIN DEMISE

Stage V TTTS can occur after expectant management or attempts at therapy. In a systematic review that included 160 monochorionic twin pregnancies, Ong and colleagues[31] found that death of one twin was associated with increased risk of preterm delivery, with 68% delivering preterm, and neurologic abnormality at 4 weeks of life, which was observed in 18% of survivors. But even with PTB notwithstanding, whenever a single monochorionic twin fetal demise occurs there is potential for surviving co-twin perinatal mortality and morbidity related to acute hypovolemia in the setting of transient hemodynamic instability and an acute intertwin exsanguination event within the shared twin placental circulation. Neurologic morbidity is a particular concern, as abrupt survivor hypotension related to a "backbleed" phenomenon can precipitate an ischemic stroke. One systematic review of cases with single twin demise in 116 monochorionic pregnancies found abnormal brain imaging in 20% of surviving twins.[32]

Despite this plausible concern, single twin survivorship after laser surgery has not been conclusively proved to confer additional risk for neurologic morbidity when compared with dual survivorship. Cavicchioni and colleagues[33] retrospectively analyzed 45 pregnancies with stage V TTTS after laser surgery. They found that 2 pregnancies resulted in miscarriage, 2 in termination due to prenatally detected brain issues, and 2 in neonatal demise. Among survivors, 89% were neurologically normal at 6 to 44 months of life. Rossi and colleagues[34] performed a systematic review of more than 800 twin pregnancies treated with SLP and found an overall 11.1% rate of neurologic morbidity. When neurologic morbidity was compared between 1 and 2 survivors, no difference was apparent (17.3% vs 18.0%, $P = .55$).

NEUROLOGIC MORBIDITY OF PREGNANCIES WITH PERSISTENT ANASTOMOSIS AFTER LASER

The aim of fetoscopic laser surgery is to functionally separate, or "dichorionize," monochorionic twin fetal circulations, ideally eliminating all intertwin residual anastomoses. In reality, complete photocoagulation of all intertwin anastomoses is often not achieved. Investigators have hypothesized that residual patent anastomosis may actually play more of a role in neurologic outcomes by precipitating recurrent TTTS, acute intertwin exsanguination, and twin anemia polycythemia sequence (TAPS).[35] One study examined placentas of 77 pregnancies treated with laser surgery for TTTS and found that residual anastomoses (RA) were found in 32% of placentas, with most located near the margin of the placenta (X). Neurologic outcomes do not seem to be associated with the presence of RA alone. Lopriore and colleagues examined 52 placentas of monochorionic pregnancies treated with laser surgery for TTTS and found similar rates of RA in 33% of placentas. There was no significant difference in adverse outcomes (defined as intrauterine fetal demise, neonatal death, or severe cerebral injury) between those with RA (18%) versus those without RA (29%, $P = .23$).[36]

Small, submillimeter-caliber intertwin anastomoses are believed to be key to the development of TAPS, which affects up to 13% of TTTS pregnancies treated with laser. Slaghekke and colleagues[37] evaluated 33 pregnancies (11% of a larger cohort) affected by TAPS after laser surgery for TTTS. Overall, they observed 80% survival and, on long-term assessment of 47 surviving children (89%) at a minimum of 2 years of age, they found major neurodevelopmental impairment (defined as CP, cognitive development score of <70 [>2 SD less than the mean], motor development score of less than 70 [>2 SD less than the mean], bilateral blindness, or bilateral deafness requiring amplification) in 9%, with mild to moderate cognitive impairment in 17%. There are insufficient data to determine if TAPS occurring after laser surgery increases risk for neurologic deficits when compared with laser surgery survivors unaffected by TAPS.

Laser photocoagulation along the vascular equator is a prophylactic adjunct procedure performed at the time of laser surgery that has been demonstrated to reduce the occurrence of postlaser TAPS and recurrent TTTS. This procedure, referred to as the Solomon technique, was evaluated in an open-label, international trial in which 274 women were randomized to either SLP with the Solomon technique or standard SLP alone. The investigators found a significant reduction in the incidence of their primary outcome (incidence of TAPS, recurrence of TTTS, perinatal mortality, or severe neonatal morbidity) occurring in 34% of the Solomon group versus 49% of the SLP group.[38] Of the 235 fetuses who survived to 2 years of age, 116 (92%) were evaluated for pediatric neurodevelopmental outcomes. The investigators found no difference in their primary outcome (survival without neurodevelopmental impairment) between Solomon and standard SLP groups (67% vs 68%, $P = .92$), nor the rate of neurodevelopmental impairment in long-term survivors (11% vs 9%, $P = .61$).[39]

NEUROIMAGING AFTER SELECTIVE LASER PHOTOCOAGULATION

Because of the angioarchitecture of the shared placenta and sudden hemodynamic shifts in TTTS, twins are at risk of cerebral ischemia, infarction, and possible reperfusion injury. In TTTS, antenatal detection of these lesions is possible even before any intervention.[40] Several types of cerebral lesions have been described: cystic periventricular leukomalacia, IVH, posthemorrhagic ventricular dilation, cerebral atrophy, and ischemic stroke.[41] Cerebral lesions can be detected on ultrasound or MRI, with both modalities frequently used together for evaluation. Vanderbilt and colleagues examined imaging from 242 "high-risk survivors" of laser therapy for TTTS, defined by delivery under 32 weeks gestational age or development of clinical indications for neuroimaging. They found that 19%[42] of fetuses showed any lesion and 7%[18] severe lesions (defined as IVH grade III–IV, cystic periventricular leukomalacia, ventriculomegaly and/or hydrocephalus, microcephaly, infarctions, porencephalic/Dandy-Walker cysts, or bilateral other cysts).[43]

Overall, studies suggest that MRI is more accurate than ultrasound at diagnosing fetal brain anomalies.[44] Malinger and colleagues retrospectively analyzed 42 pregnancies referred for intracranial anomalies that underwent neurosonographic and MRI examinations and found that MRI was better at detecting parenchymal anomalies and ventricular dilation.[45] MRI is not limited by maternal skeleton or bowel gas and does not need the presence of amniotic fluid to allow for the visualization of fetal structures. In addition, the use of diffusion-weighted imaging in MRI provides quantitative information of the tissue microstructure that can show additional destructive brain processes.[46] Although MRI is likely superior as a fetal neuroimaging modality, ultrasound remains a powerful imaging tool for neuropathology, especially when high-frequency transvaginal probes are used with 3-dimensional imaging.[42]

Regardless of the modality used, antenatal identification of neurologic morbidity is important, as it may influence management plans. Currently there is insufficient evidence to recommend when, how, or how often to image these pregnancies before or after laser surgery or other intervention for TTTS. In general, fetal MRI to assess ischemic injury is best when performed in the third trimester (Simpson 2012 AJOG). However, studies indicate that most insults are detected soon after the procedure. Weisz and colleagues[47] prospectively evaluated 30 pregnancies treated with laser surgery for TTTS. Of the 6 pregnancies with fetal neurologic insults, all had been diagnosed by MRI 1 to 5 days after procedure, with no new diagnosis on routine imaging at 30 to 32 weeks. However, in this small cohort, no patients underwent preprocedural MRI, and it is possible these neurologic insults occurred before laser surgery. Although diffusion-weighted imaging can detect ischemic and hemorrhagic brain lesions early, these changes can persist for weeks.[48] At the authors' institution, they routinely obtain fetal MRI 2 to 3 weeks after laser surgery or before 24 weeks gestational age, whichever comes first.[49–58]

SUMMARY

Pediatric neurologic outcomes overall seem superior after fetoscopic laser photocoagulation when compared with amnioreduction or expectant management for the management of TTTS. Major neurologic morbidity rates after laser surgery have been reported in several series, with results ranging from as low as 4% to as high as 18%, with most of the reviews revealing rates less than 10%. Earlier gestational age at birth, low birthweight, and higher stage of twin-twin transfusion at diagnosis may be associated with poorer neurologic outcomes after laser therapy. When intracranial insults are detected prenatally, it is not always clear when they occurred, as preprocedural fetal MRI is not a routine practice.

CLINICS CARE POINTS

- Although there is currently clinical equipoise regarding the optimal management of stage I disease, it is widely accepted that intervention is recommended for stage II to IV TTTS due to a substantial risk of perinatal morbidity and mortality with untreated early onset advanced-stage TTTS.
- Fetoscopic laser therapy is considered superior treatment to amnioreduction as it has been associated with improved survival and lower rates of neurological morbidity; as the procedure has aged, overall survival has improved.
- While data on neurologic morbidity after amnioreduction is limited, it appears that fetoscopic laser surgery carries lower rates of morbidity.
- Major neurologic morbidity rates after laser surgery have been reported as low as 4% to as high as 18%, with most reviews revealing rates under 10%.
- The literature seems to indicate that donors and recipients are at equal risk for cerebral injury after laser surgery, however this is based on secondary outcomes of potentially underpowered studies.
- Advanced Quintero staging has been associated with poorer immediate outcomes such as perinatal mortality and morbidity, as well as long-term neuromorbidity.
- A survival benefit among dual versus single twin survivors after laser surgery has not been conclusively proven in the literature.

DISCLOSURE

R.S. Miller disclosed receiving honorarium for writing a article on TRAP sequence for UpToDate. D. Sutton has no disclosures.

REFERENCES

1. Hamilton BE, Martin JA, Osterman MJ, et al. Births: final data for 2014. Natl Vital Stat Rep 2015;64:1.
2. Cameron AH, Edwards JH, Derom R, et al. The value of twin surveys in the study of malformations. Eur J Obstet Gynecol Reprod Biol 1983;14:347.
3. Ananth CV, Chauhan SP. Epidemiology of twinning in developed countries. Semin Perinatol 2012;36(3):156–61.
4. Lee YM, Wylie BJ, Simpson LL, et al. Twin chorionicity and the risk of stillbirth. Obstet Gynecol 2008;111:301.
5. Leduc L, Takser L, Rinfret D. Persistence of adverse obstetric and neonatal outcomes in monochorionic twins after exclusion of disorders unique to monochorionic placentation. Am J Obstet Gynecol 2005;193:1670–5.
6. Roberts D, Neilson JP, Kilby MD, et al. Interventions for the treatment of twin-twin transfusion syndrome. Cochrane Database Syst Rev 2014;(1):CD002073.
7. Society for Maternal-Fetal Medicine, Simpson LL. Twin-twin transfusion syndrome. Am J Obstet Gynecol 2013;208:3.
8. Bajoria R, Ward S, Sooranna SR. Influence of vasopressin in the pathogenesis of oligohydramnios-polyhydramnios in monochorionic twins. Eur J Obstet Gynecol Reprod Biol 2004;113:49.
9. Mahieu-Caputo D, Dommergues M, Delezoide AL, et al. Twin-to-twin transfusion syndrome. Role of the fetal renin-angiotensin system. Am J Pathol 2000;156:629.
10. Quintero RA, Morales WJ, Allen MH, et al. Staging of twin-twin transfusion syndrome. J Perinatol 1999;19:550.
11. Bower SJ, Flack NJ, Sepulveda W, et al. Uterine artery blood flow response to correction of amniotic fluid volume. Am J Obstet Gynecol 1995;173(2):502–7.
12. Mari G, Roberts A, Detti L, et al. Perinatal morbidity and mortality rates in severe twin-twin transfusion syndrome: results of the International Amnioreduction Registry. Am J Obstet Gynecol 2001;185(3):708–15.
13. De Lia JE, Cruikshank DP, Keye WR Jr. Fetoscopic neodymium:YAG laser occlusion of placental vessels in severe twin-twin transfusion syndrome. Obstet Gynecol 1990;75(6):1046–53.
14. Crombleholme TM, Shera D, Lee H, et al. A prospective, randomized, multicenter trial of amnioreduction vs selective fetoscopic laser photocoagulation for the treatment of severe twin-twin transfusion syndrome. Am J Obstet Gynecol 2007;197(4):396.e1-9.
15. Akkermans J, Peeters SH, Klumper FJ, et al. Twenty-five years of fetoscopic laser coagulation in twin-twin transfusion syndrome: a systematic review. Fetal Diagn Ther 2015;38(4):241–53.
16. Scher AI, Petterson B, Blair E, et al. The risk of mortality or cerebral palsy in twins: a collaborative population-based study. Pediatr Res 2002;52(5):671–81.
17. Li X, Morokuma S, Fukushima K, et al. Prognosis and long-term neurodevelopmental outcome in conservatively treated twin-to-twin transfusion syndrome. BMC Pregnancy Childbirth 2011;11:32.
18. Reisner DP, Mahony BS, Petty CN, et al. Stuck twin syndrome: outcome in thirty-seven consecutive cases. Am J Obstet Gynecol 1993;169:991–5.
19. Graef C, Ellenrieder B, Hecher K, et al. Long-term neurodevelopmental outcome of 167 children after intrauterine laser treatment for severe twin-twin transfusion syndrome. Am J Obstet Gynecol 2006;194(2):303–8.

20. Hecher K, Gardiner HM, Diemert A, et al. Long-term outcomes for monochorionic twins after laser therapy in twin-to-twin transfusion syndrome. Lancet Child Adolesc Health 2018;2(7):525–35.

21. Spruijt M, Steggerda S, Rath M, et al. Cerebral injury in twin-twin transfusion syndrome treated with fetoscopic laser surgery. Obstet Gynecol 2012;120(1):15–20.

22. Vohr BR, Stephens BE, Higgins RD, et al. Are outcomes of extremely preterm infants improving? Impact of Bayley assessment on outcomes. J Pediatr 2012; 161(2):222–8.e3.

23. Spruijt MS, Lopriore E, Tan RNGB, et al. Long-term neurodevelopmental outcome in twin-to-twin transfusion syndrome: is there still room for improvement? J Clin Med 2019;8(8):1226.

24. van Klink JM, Koopman HM, Rijken M, et al. Long-term neurodevelopmental outcome in survivors of twin-to-twin transfusion syndrome. Twin Res Hum Genet 2016;19(3):255–61.

25. van Klink JM, Koopman HM, van Zwet EW, et al. Cerebral injury and neurodevelopmental impairment after amnioreduction versus laser surgery in twin-twin transfusion syndrome: a systematic review and meta-analysis. Fetal Diagn Ther 2013;33(2):81–9.

26. Miller V. Neonatal cerebral infarction. Semin Pediatr Neurol 2000;7:278–88.

27. Rossi AC, D'Addario V. Comparison of donor and recipient outcomes following laser therapy performed for twin-twin transfusion syndrome: a meta-analysis and review of literature. Am J Perinatol 2009;26(1):27–32.

28. Senat MV, Deprest J, Boulvain M, et al. Endoscopic laser surgery versus serial amnioreduction for severe twin-to-twin transfusion syndrome. N Engl J Med 2004;351(2):136–44.

29. Lopriore E, Ortibus E, Acosta-Rojas R, et al. Risk factors for neurodevelopment impairment in twin-twin transfusion syndrome treated with fetoscopic laser surgery. Obstet Gynecol 2009;113(2 Pt 1):361–6.

30. Gray PH, Poulsen L, Gilshenan K, et al. Neurodevelopmental outcome and risk factors for disability for twin-twin transfusion syndrome treated with laser surgery. Am J Obstet Gynecol 2011;204(2):159.e1-6.

31. Ong SS, Zamora J, Khan KS, et al. Prognosis for the co-twin following single-twin death: a systematic review. BJOG 2006;113(9):992–8.

32. Mackie FL, Rigby A, Morris RK, et al. Prognosis of the co-twin following spontaneous single intrauterine fetal death in twin pregnancies: a systematic review and meta-analysis. BJOG 2019;126(5):569–78.

33. Cavicchioni O, Yamamoto M, Robyr R, et al. Intrauterine fetal demise following laser treatment in twin-to-twin transfusion syndrome. BJOG 2006;113(5):590–4.

34. Rossi AC, Vanderbilt D, Chmait RH. Neurodevelopmental outcomes after laser therapy for twin-twin transfusion syndrome: a systematic review and meta-analysis. Obstet Gynecol 2011;118(5):1145–50.

35. De Lia JE, Worthington D. Re: "Comparison of donor and recipient outcomes following laser therapy performed for twin-twin transfusion syndrome: a meta-analysis and review of literature. Am J Perinatol 2009;26(1):27-32". Am J Perinatol 2009;26(8):613–5.

36. Stirnemann J, Chalouhi G, Essaoui M, et al. Fetal brain imaging following laser surgery in twin-to-twin surgery. BJOG 2018;125(9):1186–91.

37. Slaghekke F, van Klink JM, Koopman HM, et al. Neurodevelopmental outcome in twin anemia-polycythemia sequence after laser surgery for twin-twin transfusion syndrome. Ultrasound Obstet Gynecol 2014;44(3):316–21.

38. Slaghekke F, Lopriore E, Lewi L, et al. Fetoscopic laser coagulation of the vascular equator versus selective coagulation for twin-to-twin transfusion syndrome: an open-label randomised controlled trial. Lancet 2014;383(9935):2144–51.

39. van Klink JM, Slaghekke F, Balestriero MA, et al. Neurodevelopmental outcome at 2 years in twin-twin transfusion syndrome survivors randomized for the Solomon trial. Am J Obstet Gynecol 2016;214(1):113.e1-7.

40. Bejar R, Vigliocco G, Gramajo H, et al. Antenatal origin of neurologic damage in newborn infants. II. Multiple gestations. Am J Obstet Gynecol 1990;162:1230–6.

41. Spruijt MS, Lopriore E, Steggerda SJ, et al. Twin-twin transfusion syndrome in the era of fetoscopic laser surgery: antenatal management, neonatal outcome and beyond. Expert Rev Hematol 2020;13(3):259–67.

42. Monteagudo A, Timor-Tritsch IE, Mayberry P. Three-dimensional transvaginal neurosonography of the fetal brain: 'navigating' in the volume scan. Ultrasound Obstet Gynecol 2000;16(4):307–13.

43. Vanderbilt DL, Schrager SM, Llanes A, et al. Prevalence and risk factors of cerebral lesions in neonates after laser surgery for twin-twin transfusion syndrome. Am J Obstet Gynecol 2012;207(4):320.e1-6.

44. Hart AR, Embleton ND, Bradburn M, et al. Accuracy of in-utero MRI to detect fetal brain abnormalities and prognosticate developmental outcome: postnatal follow-up of the MERIDIAN cohort. Lancet Child Adolesc Health 2020;4(2):131–40.

45. Malinger G, Ben-Sira L, Lev D, et al. Fetal brain imaging: a comparison between magnetic resonance imaging and dedicated neurosonography. Ultrasound Obstet Gynecol 2004;23(4):333–40.

46. Mailath-Pokorny M, Kasprian G, Mitter C, et al. Magnetic resonance methods in fetal neurology. Semin Fetal Neonatal Med 2012;17(5):278–84.

47. Weisz B, Hoffmann C, Ben-Baruch S, et al. Early detection by diffusion-weighted sequence magnetic resonance imaging of severe brain lesions after fetoscopic laser coagulation for twin-twin transfusion syndrome. Ultrasound Obstet Gynecol 2014;44(1):44–9.

48. Tarui T, Khwaja OS, Estroff JA, et al. Fetal MR imaging evidence of prolonged apparent diffusion coefficient decrease in fetal death. AJNR Am J Neuroradiol 2011;32(7):E126–8.

49. Sutcliffe AG, Sebire NJ, Pigott AJ, et al. Outcome for children born after in utero lacor ablation therapy for severe twin-to-twin transfusion syndrome. BJOG 2001;108(12):1246–50.

50. Banek CS, Hecher K, Hackeloer BJ, et al. Long-term neurodevelopmental outcome after intrauterine laser treatment for severe twin-twin transfusion syndrome. Am J Obstet Gynecol 2003;188(4):876–80.

51. Lopriore E, Middeldorp JM, Sueters M, et al. Long-term neurodevelopmental outcome in twin-to-twin transfusion syndrome treated with fetoscopic laser surgery. Am J Obstet Gynecol 2007;196(3):231.e1-4.

52. Lenclen R, Ciarlo G, Paupe A, et al. Neurodevelopmental outcome at 2 years in children born preterm treated by amnioreduction or fetoscopic laser surgery for twin-to-twin transfusion syndrome: comparison with dichorionic twins. Am J Obstet Gynecol 2009;201(3):291.e1-5.

53. Salomon LJ, Ortqvist L, Aegerter P, et al. Long-term developmental follow-up of infants who participated in a randomized clinical trial of amniocentesis vs laser photocoagulation for the treatment of twin-to-twin transfusion syndrome. Am J Obstet Gynecol 2010;203(5):444.e1-7.

54. Graeve P, Banek C, Stegmann-Woessner G, et al. Neurodevelopmental outcome at 6 years of age after intrauterine laser therapy for twin-twin transfusion syndrome. Acta Paediatr 2012;101(12):1200–5.
55. Chang YL, Chao AS, Chang SD, et al. The neurological outcomes of surviving twins in severe twin-twin transfusion syndrome treated by fetoscopic laser photocoagulation at a newly established center. Prenat Diagn 2012;32(9):893–6.
56. Vanderbilt DL, Schrager SM, Llanes A, et al. Predictors of 2-year cognitive performance after laser surgery for twin-twin transfusion syndrome. Am J Obstet Gynecol 2014;211(4):388.e1-7.
57. McIntosh J, Meriki N, Joshi A, et al. Long term developmental outcomes of preschool age children following laser surgery for twin-to-twin transfusion syndrome. Early Hum Dev 2014;90(12):837–42.
58. van Klink JM, Koopman HM, van Zwet EW, et al. Improvement in neurodevelopmental outcome in survivors of twin-twin transfusion syndrome treated with laser surgery. Am J Obstet Gynecol 2014;210(6):540.e1-7.

An Update on Biologic Agents During Pregnancy

Ibrahim Hammad, MD, MSCI*, T. Flint Porter, MD

KEYWORDS

- Immunosuppressive agents • Pregnancy • Autoimmune disease • Adverse effects

KEY POINTS

- Most biological agents are safe to use in pregnancy with little to risk for teratogenicity or complications in pregnancy.
- Treatment options should be individualized to the patient's disease activity, response to medication, and maternal risks.
- Data gathering needs to continue in order to obtain a more complete profile for each of the categories of medication used.

INTRODUCTION

It is often necessary to continue immunosuppressive agents during pregnancy in women with pre-existing autoimmune disease (**Table 1**). Some of the most frequently prescribed immunosuppressive agents may be used safely during pregnancy, while others are strictly contraindicated. As with any drug during pregnancy, the goal of auto-immune treatment is to adequately control disease activity without placing the undue risk on the mother and fetus. The decision to use any biologic agents during pregnancy should be based on the clinical context, risks associated with individual medications, and the stage of pregnancy. In this article, the biologic agents have been divided into 4 categories: minimal risk, uncertain risk, moderate risk, and high risk.

BIOLOGIC AGENTS WITH MINIMAL RISK
Hydroxychloroquine

Substantial experience suggests that antimalarial drugs, such as hydroxychloroquine, may be used safely for the treatment of systemic lupus erythematosus (SLE) during pregnancy.[1-4] Previous concerns about teratogenicity, including ototoxicity[5] and eye damage,[6] have been largely dismissed. The findings of a case-control trial that

Maternal-Fetal Medicine, Intermountain Healthcare, and the University of Utah, 5121 S Cottonwood Street, Ste 100, Murray, UT 84115, USA
* Corresponding author.
E-mail address: Ibrahim.hammad@imail.org

Clin Perinatol 47 (2020) 733–742
https://doi.org/10.1016/j.clp.2020.08.003
0095-5108/20/© 2020 Elsevier Inc. All rights reserved.

Table 1
Biologic agents during pregnancy

Class	Obstetric Complications	Comments
Minimal risk		
Hydroxychloroquine	None reported	More effective than glucocorticoids in flare prevention during pregnancy
Glucocorticoids	Increase risk for diabetes, hypertension, preeclampsia, PPROM, IURG	Patients requiring chronic maintenance therapy are best treated with prednisolone or methylprednisolone
Sulfasalazine	None reported	Folic acid supplementation recommended before attempting pregnancy
Nonsteroidal Anti-inflammatory	Intraventricular hemorrhage, necrotizing enterocolitis, periventricular leukomalacia, oligohydramnios, closure of fetal ductus arteriosus.	Chronic usage should be avoided
Azathioprine	Preterm birth and IUGR	
Cyclosporine A	A rise in maternal creatinine and an increase in preterm birth and small for gestational age infants	
Uncertain risk		
TNF-α inhibitors	None reported	Concerns about an association between TNF-α inhibitors and fetal VACTERL, but large database suggested no increase compared with the general population
Moderate risk		
Cyclophosphamide	None reported	Use in the second and third trimesters has not been associated with adverse perinatal outcomes
Rituximab	Spontaneous abortion and preterm birth	Neonatal B-cell lymphocytopenia that persists for several months
Belimumab	Unknown	Little is known about its impact on maternal or fetal outcomes

(*continued on next page*)

Table 1 (*continued*)		
Class	Obstetric Complications	Comments
High risk		
Methotrexate	Spontaneous abortion, cranial-facial anomalies, limb reduction defects, congenital heart disease, and neurodevelopmental delay, IUGR	Pregnancy should delay conception for at least 3 menstrual cycles after discontinuation of methotrexate
MMF	Cleft lip and palate, micrognathia, microtia, and auditory canal abnormalities, IUGR	Conception should be delayed at least 6 weeks after discontinuing MMF
Leflunomide	Multiple major and minor fetal anomalies	Remains detectable for up to 2 years after drug discontinuation

Abbreviations: IUGR, intrauterine fetal growth restriction; PPROM, preterm prelabor rupture of membranes; VACTERL, vertebral anomalies, anal atresia, cardiac defects, tracheoesophageal fistula, esophageal atresia, renal anomalies, and limb dysplasia.

assessed the effects of in utero exposure to hydroxychloroquine are reassuring.[4] The authors reported no differences between 122 infants with in utero exposure to hydroxychloroquine and 70 control infants in the number and type of defects identified at birth or in the proportion of infants with visual, hearing, growth, or developmental abnormalities at follow-up (median 24 months). Hydroxychloroquine may be more effective than glucocorticoids in flare prevention during pregnancy. In a randomized controlled trial, women who continued hydroxychloroquine during pregnancy experienced a significant reduction in SLE disease activity compared with women who changed to glucocorticoid therapy.[7]

Glucocorticoids

The drugs most commonly given to pregnant women with autoimmune disease are glucocorticoid preparations, both as maintenance therapy and in bursts to treat suspected disease exacerbation. The doses used in pregnancy are the same as those used in nonpregnant patients. Pregnancy per se is not an indication to reduce the dose of glucocorticoids. However, a carefully monitored reduction in dosage may be reasonable in appropriately selected women whose disease appears to be in remission.

Although glucocorticoids have a low potential for teratogenesis, they are not without risk during pregnancy. Patients requiring chronic maintenance therapy are best treated with prednisolone or methylprednisolone because of their conversion to relatively inactive forms by the abundance of 11β-hydroxysteroid dehydrogenase found in the human placenta. Glucocorticoids with fluorine at the 9-α position (eg, dexamethasone and betamethasone) are considerably less well metabolized by the placenta, and chronic use during pregnancy should be avoided, because both have been associated with fetal adverse effects, more specifically, fetal weight reduction.[8] Maternal adverse effects of chronic glucocorticoid therapy are the same as in nonpregnant patients and include weight gain, striae, acne, hirsutism, immunosuppression, osteonecrosis, and gastrointestinal ulceration. During pregnancy, chronic glucocorticoid therapy has also been associated with an increased risk of preeclampsia, uteroplacental insufficiency, preterm rupture of membranes, intrauterine growth restriction (IUGR), and glucose intolerance.[9–12] Women undergoing chronic treatment with glucocorticoids should be screened for gestational diabetes at the beginning of each trimester.

Sulfasalazine

Sulfasalazine is a combination of salicylate and a sulfa antibiotic that possesses anti-inflammatory properties. It is used in pregnancy most commonly for patients with inflammatory bowel disease. Both sulfasalazine and its metabolite, sulfapyridine, cross the placenta. Even so, large studies have found no teratogenic effect.[13] Its mechanism of action involves inhibition of dihydrofolate reductase inhibitor, an action that theoretically increases the risk of neural tube defects. Whether increasing the dose of folic acid supplementation before pregnancy decreases that risk is unknown. However, women taking sulfasalazine who are considering pregnancy should take the minimum recommended dose of 0.4 mg.

Nonsteroidal Anti-inflammatory Drugs

Nonsteroidal anti-inflammatory drugs (NSAIDs) are used most frequently outside of pregnancy because of their analgesic, anti-inflammatory, and anti-platelet properties. All NSAID medications readily cross the placenta, and their use during pregnancy depends on gestational age, the specific drug, and dosage. First-trimester exposure to NSAID medication has not been associated with an increased risk for congenital malformation or perinatal mortality.[14] Likewise, no adverse effects have been identified with low-dose aspirin (81 mg) use throughout pregnancy, sometimes recommended for women with a history of preeclampsia.[15,16] However, the use of regular-dose aspirin (325 mg) and other NSAIDs later in pregnancy has been associated with several untoward fetal effects; these include intraventricular hemorrhage, necrotizing enterocolitis, and periventricular leukomalacia.[17,18] Short-term tocolytic therapy with indomethacin appears to be safe,[19,20] but when used after 32 weeks may result in constriction or closure of the fetal ductus arteriosus.[17] Long-term use of all NSAIDs has been associated with decreased fetal urine output and oligohydramnios, as well as neonatal renal insufficiency.[21,22] Given these risks, chronic use of adult dosages of aspirin and other NSAIDs should be avoided during pregnancy, especially after the first trimester. Acetaminophen and narcotic-containing preparations are acceptable alternatives if analgesia is needed during pregnancy.

Azathioprine

Limited data suggest that azathioprine, a derivative of 6-mercaptopurine, is not a teratogen in people,[23,24] although it has been associated with preterm birth and intrauterine growth restriction.[25–27] Women who require azathioprine to control SLE disease activity should not necessarily be discouraged from becoming pregnant. However, potential fetal risks should be carefully weighed against the benefits of the medication.

Cyclosporine A

The immunosuppressive action of cyclosporine A works through the inhibition of the production and release of interleukin (IL)-2. Its use during pregnancy is limited to the treatment of lupus nephritis and severe arthritis. Only a small amount is transferred via the placenta into the fetal circulation, and experience from studies in organ transplant patients indicates a low risk of teratogenicity.[28] Cyclosporine A has been associated with a rise in maternal creatinine and an increase in preterm birth and small for gestational age infants.[20]

BIOLOGIC AGENTS WITH UNCERTAIN RISK

Experience with the use of these medications during pregnancy is limited. However, emerging data suggest minimal risk.

Tumor Necrosis Factor-α Inhibitors

Tumor necrosis factor-α (TNF-α) inhibition results in an increase in circulating T regulatory cells and a restored capacity to inhibit cytokine production.[29] They are currently used as maintenance medications for autoimmune disease. This category of drugs includes infliximab, etanercept, adalimumab, certolizumab, and golimumab. They are all transferred across the placenta, with the exception of certolizumab.

Animal studies using infliximab,[30] adalimumab,[31] and certolizumab[32] have not reported an increase in the rate of teratogenic effects. Concerns about an association between TNF-α inhibitors and fetal VACTERL (vertebral anomalies, anal atresia, cardiac defects, tracheoesophageal fistula, esophageal atresia, renal anomalies, and limb dysplasia) syndrome were raised in early series.[33] However, data from a large European congenital malformation database reported no increase in VACTERL anomalies in infants exposed in utero to TNF inhibitors compared with the general population.[34] Experience with hundreds of pregnancies exposed to anti-TNF-α agents also suggests that TNF-α inhibitors are not teratogenic and not associated with obstetric complications.[35,36] Proceedings of the American College of Rheumatology Reproductive Health Summit[37] stated that although data were somewhat limited, "TNF inhibitors are considered to be compatible with pregnancy."

BIOLOGIC AGENTS WITH MODERATE RISK

The use of the following agents during pregnancy should be individualized. They pose a moderate risk during pregnancy but may be necessary when an active maternal disease cannot be adequately controlled otherwise.

Cyclophosphamide

Cyclophosphamide has been reported to be teratogenic in both animal[38] and human studies[39,40] and should be avoided during the first trimester. Although data are limited, cyclophosphamide use in the second and third trimesters has not been associated with adverse perinatal outcomes.[41,42] Even so, its use should be limited to circumstances wherein the benefits clearly outweigh the potential risks, such as severe progressive proliferative glomerulonephritis refractory to immunosuppressive agents with better safety profiles.

Rituximab

Rituximab is a humanized monoclonal antibody that targets the CD20 antigen on pre-B and mature B lymphocytes to cause cell lysis and depletion. Although the manufacturer recommends discontinuing rituximab 1 year before conception, published case reports, systematic reviews, and case series of its use during early pregnancy are reassuring.[43,44] The authors identified over 100 pregnancies exposed to rituximab; approximately 12% had a spontaneous abortion, and 41% delivered before 37 weeks. With that being said, the limitations of these studies are their retrospective nature and small size of the case series and reports, the potential under-reporting, and lack of information on potential confounders. Rituximab crosses the placenta, and when given in the third trimester has been associated with neonatal B-cell lymphocytopenia that persists for several months.[45]

Belimumab

Belimumab is a monoclonal antibody that inhibits B lymphocyte stimulation. Little is known about its impact on maternal or fetal outcomes, and it would seem prudent to avoid its use during pregnancy and breastfeeding. The manufacturer advises avoiding conception for 4 months after discontinuing the drug.

BIOLOGIC AGENTS WITH HIGH-RISK

These medications are contraindicated during pregnancy because of teratogenic and/or abortion risks. Reproductive-aged women using these medications to control their autoimmune conditions should be counseled against pregnancy. They should be on a highly effective birth control method unless their disease can be adequately controlled on another regimen.

METHOTREXATE

Methotrexate is commonly used to provide long-term maintenance immunosuppression in patients with autoimmune conditions. It is a folate antagonist that is abortogenic and teratogenic when used in early pregnancy. It has been associated with cranial-facial anomalies, limb reduction defects, congenital heart disease, and neurodevelopmental delay, mainly when used before 10 weeks.[21,46–48] Methotrexate is widely distributed in maternal tissues and may persist for up to 4 months in the liver. Those considering pregnancy should delay conception for at least 3 menstrual cycles after discontinuation of methotrexate. If pregnancy occurs while on methotrexate, these women should be counseled about the previously noted effects; if continuing pregnancy is elected, then a level 2 ultrasonography, a fetal echocardiogram, and interval growth ultrasounds should be considered.

Mycophenolate

Mycophenolate (MMF) works by inhibition of purine biosynthesis and is frequently used in patients with lupus nephritis as maintenance therapy. Its use decreases the need for high-dose steroids and cyclophosphamide. Like methotrexate, MMF is abortogenic and teratogenic and has been associated with cleft lip and palate, micrognathia, microtia, and auditory canal abnormalities.[49,50] Conception should be delayed at least 6 weeks after discontinuing MMF.

Leflunomide

Leflunomide is used in the treatment of inflammatory arthritis and lupus-related skin manifestations. It works by inhibition of dihydroorotate dehydrogenase, an enzyme necessary for pyrimidine biosynthesis. It is a teratogen associated with major and minor anomalies.[51] Its metabolite (teriflunomide) is widely distributed and remains detectable for up to 2 years after drug discontinuation. Pregnancy should be avoided until serum drug levels are less than 0.02 mg/L on 2 tests performed 2 weeks apart. Cholestyramine (8 g orally 3 times daily for 11 days) may be used to augment drug elimination.

OTHER IMMUNOMODULATORS

Several immunomodulators either have not been studied in human pregnancy or have been associated with congenital anomalies in animal studies. Tocilizumab is a humanized monoclonal antibody directed against the IL-6 receptor. Administration of tocilizumab to cynomolgus monkeys during organogenesis is reported to cause embryonic or fetal death and abortion at doses just above those used in people. Anakinra is a recombinant IL-1 receptor antagonist, and although studies in pregnant rats are reassuring, its use in human pregnancy or breastfeeding has not been reported. Abatacept is a recombinant fusion protein that selectively modulates T cell activation. Like tocilizumab and anakinra, its safety in pregnancy is uncertain. Until further information is available, none of these medications should be used during pregnancy, and conception should be delayed for at least 2 to 3 months after discontinuation.

SUMMARY

The use of immunosuppressive biologic agents is continuously increasing, as they have proven to be effective in the treatment of many diseases. Most agents are safe to use in pregnancy, with little to no risk for teratogenicity or pregnancy-related complication. However, some of the agents are contraindicated. When pregnancy is being considered or has occurred, women on biologic agents should be counseled about the possible effects of the medication. Furthermore, an individualized approach should be undertaken, where the risks of untreated disease and the adverse effects on the pregnancy are in the balance of decision making.

CLINICS CARE POINTS

- The use of *Hydroxychloroquine, Sulfasalazine, Azathioprine, Cyclosporine A*, low dose *Aspirin* is considered safe in pregnancy.
- The use of Glucocorticoids in pregnancy is safe, however, there is an increased risk for gestational diabetes and pregnancy induced hypertension.
- NSAID used in the first trimester or for a short period in the second trimester does not seem to be increasing the risk toward the pregnancy. They should be avoided in the third trimester.
- TNF-α inhibitors appear to be safe in pregnancy, however, data continues to emerge.
- The use of *Cyclophosphamide, Rituximab, and Belimumab* should be limited only in cases where other agents are not available and where the benefits outweigh the risks.
- *Methotrexate, Mycophenolate, and Leflunomide* should not be used in pregnancy. Preconception counseling is recommended to assess options for changing medications or timing of pregnancy.

REFERENCES

1. Buchanan NM, Toubi E, Khamashta MA, et al. Hydroxychloroquine and lupus pregnancy: review of a series of 36 cases. Ann Rheum Dis 1996;55(7):486–8.

2. Khamashta MA, Buchanan NM, Hughes GR. The use of hydroxychloroquine in lupus pregnancy: the British experience. Lupus 1996;5(Suppl 1):S65–6.

3. Motta M, Tincani A, Faden D, et al. Antimalarial agents in pregnancy. Lancet 2002;359(9305):524–5.

4. Costedoat-Chalumeau N, Amoura Z, Duhaut P, et al. Safety of hydroxychloroquine in pregnant patients with connective tissue diseases: a study of one hundred thirty-three cases compared with a control group. Arthritis Rheum 2003; 48(11):3207–11.

5. Hart CW, Naunton RF. The ototoxicity of chloroquine phosphate. Arch Otolaryngol 1964;80:407–12.

6. Nylander U. Ocular damage in chloroquine therapy. Acta Ophthalmol 1967;(Suppl 92):1–71.

7. Levy RA, Vilela VS, Cataldo MJ, et al. Hydroxychloroquine (HCQ) in lupus pregnancy: double-blind and placebo-controlled study. Lupus 2001;10(6):401–4.

8. Wapner RJ, Sorokin Y, Thom EA, et al. Single versus weekly courses of antenatal corticosteroids: evaluation of safety and efficacy. National Institute of Child Health and human development maternal fetal medicine units network. Am J Obstet Gynecol 2006;195:633–42.

9. Lockshin MD, Qamar T, Druzin ML. Hazards of lupus pregnancy. J Rheumatol Suppl 1987;14(Suppl 13):214–7.

10. Rahman P, Gladman DD, Urowitz MB. Clinical predictors of fetal outcome in systemic lupus erythematosus. J Rheumatol 1998;25(8):1526–30.

11. Guller S, Kong L, Wozniak R, et al. Reduction of extracellular matrix protein expression in human amnion epithelial cells by glucocorticoids: a potential role in preterm rupture of the fetal membranes. J Clin Endocrinol Metab 1995;80(7):2244–50.

12. Lockwood CJ, Radunovic N, Nastic D, et al. Corticotropin-releasing hormone and related pituitary-adrenal axis hormones in fetal and maternal blood during the second half of pregnancy. J Perinat Med 1996;24(3):243–51.

13. Viktil KK, Engeland A, Furu K. Outcomes after anti-rheumatic drug use before and during pregnancy: a cohort study among 150,000 pregnant women and expectant fathers. Scand J Rheumatol 2012;41(3):196–201.

14. Daniel S, Matok I, Gorodischer R, et al. Major malformations following exposure to nonsteroidal anti-inflammatory drugs during the first trimester of pregnancy. J Rheumatol 2012;39(11):2163–9.

15. Schisterman EF, Silver RM, Lesher LL, et al. Preconception low-dose aspirin and pregnancy outcomes: results from the EAGeR randomised trial. Lancet 2014;384(9937):29–36.

16. Askie LM, Duley L, Henderson-Smart DJ, et al. Anti-platelet agents for prevention of preeclampsia: a meta-analysis of individual patient data. Lancet 2007;369(9575):1791–8.

17. Hammers AL, Sanchez-Ramos L, Kaunitz AM. Antenatal exposure to indomethacin increases the risk of severe intraventricular hemorrhage, necrotizing enterocolitis, and periventricular leukomalacia: a systematic review with metaanalysis. Am J Obstet Gynecol 2015;212(4):505.e1-13.

18. Koren G, Florescu A, Costei AM, et al. Nonsteroidal anti-inflammatory drugs during third trimester and the risk of premature closure of the ductus arteriosus: a meta-analysis. Ann Pharmacother 2006;40(5):824–9.

19. Macones GA, Robinson CA. Is there justification for using indomethacin in preterm labor? An analysis of neonatal risks and benefits. Am J Obstet Gynecol 1997;177(4):819–24.

20. Macones GA, Marder SJ, Clothier B, et al. The controversy surrounding indomethacin for tocolysis. Am J Obstet Gynecol 2001;184(3):264–72.

21. Ostensen M, Khamashta M, Lockshin M, et al. Anti-inflammatory and immunosuppressive drugs and reproduction. Arthritis Res Ther 2006;8(3):209.

22. Ostensen MVP. Nonsteroidal anti-inflammatory drugs in systemic lupus erythematosus. Lupus 2001;10:135–139. Lupus 2001;10:135–9.

23. Moskovitz DN, Bodian C, Chapman ML, et al. The effect on the fetus of medications used to treat pregnant inflammatory bowel-disease patients. Am J Gastroenterol 2004;99(4):656–61.

24. Francella A, Dyan A, Bodian C, et al. The Safety of 6-mercaptopurine for childbearing patients with inflammatory bowel disease: a retrospective cohort study. Gastroenterology 2003;124(1):9–17.

25. Armenti VT, Coscia LA, McGrory CH, et al. National transplantation pregnancy registry. Update on pregnancy and renal transplantation. Nephrol News Issues 1998;12(8):19–23.

26. Armenti VT, Moritz MJ, Davison JM. Drug safety issues in pregnancy following transplantation and immunosuppression: effects and outcomes. Drug Safety 1998;19(3):219–32.

27. Norgard B, Pedersen L, Christensen LA, et al. Therapeutic drug use in women with Crohn's disease and birth outcomes: a Danish nationwide cohort study. Am J Gastroenterol 2007;102(7):1406–13.

28. Bar Oz B, Hackman R, Einarson T, et al. Pregnancy outcome after cyclosporine therapy during pregnancy: a meta-analysis. Transplantation 2001;71(8):1051–5.

29. Ehrenstein MR, Evans JG, Singh A, et al. Compromised function of regulatory T cells in rheumatoid arthritis and reversal by anti-TNFalpha therapy. J Exp Med 2004;200(3):277–85.

30. Rychly DJ, DiPiro JT. Infections associated with tumor necrosis factor-alpha antagonists. Pharmacotherapy 2005;25(9):1181–92.

31. Baker DE. Adalimumab: human recombinant immunoglobulin g1 anti-tumor necrosis factor monoclonal antibody. Rev Gastroenterol Disord 2004;4(4):196–210.

32. Mahadevan U. Pregnancy and inflammatory bowel disease. Gastroenterol Clin North Am 2009;38(4):629–49.

33. Carter JD, Ladhani A, Ricca LR, et al. A safety assessment of tumor necrosis factor antagonists during pregnancy: a review of the Food and Drug Administration database. J Rheumatol 2009;36(3):635–41.

34. Crijns HJ, Jentink J, Garne E, et al. The distribution of congenital anomalies within the VACTERL association among tumor necrosis factor antagonist-exposed pregnancies is similar to the general population. J Rheumatol 2011;38(9):1871–4.

35. Gisbert JP, Chaparro M. Safety of anti-TNF agents during pregnancy and breastfeeding in women with inflammatory bowel disease. Am J Gastroenterol 2013;108(9):1426–38.

36. Clowse M, Wolf D, Forger F, et al. Retrospective analysis of certolizumab pegol use during pregnancy: update of impact on birth outcomes. Arthritis Rheum 2013;65:S187–8.

37. Kavanaugh A, Cush JJ, Ahmed MS, et al. Proceedings from the American College of Rheumatology Reproductive Health Summit: the management of fertility, pregnancy, and lactation in women with autoimmune and systemic inflammatory diseases. Arthritis Care Res (Hoboken) 2015;67(3):313–25.

38. Ujhazy E, Balonova T, Durisova M, et al. Teratogenicity of cyclophosphamide in New Zealand white rabbits. Neoplasma 1993;40(1):45–9.

39. Kirshon B, Wasserstrum N, Willis R, et al. Teratogenic effects of first-trimester cyclophosphamide therapy. Obstet Gynecol 1988;72(3 Pt 2):462–4.

40. Enns GM, Roeder E, Chan RT, et al. Apparent cyclophosphamide (cytoxan) embryopathy: a distinct phenotype? Am J Med Genet 1999;86(3):237–41.

41. Berry DL, Theriault RL, Holmes FA, et al. Management of breast cancer during pregnancy using a standardized protocol. J Clin Oncol 1999;17(3):855–61.

42. Ring AE, Smith IE, Jones A, et al. Chemotherapy for breast cancer during pregnancy: an 18-year experience from five London teaching hospitals. J Clin Oncol 2005;23(18):4192–7.

43. Herold M, Schnohr S, Bittrich H. Efficacy and Safety of a combined rituximab chemotherapy during pregnancy. J Clin Oncol 2001;19(14):3439.

44. Das G, Damotte V, Gelfand JM, et al. Rituximab before and during pregnancy: a systematic review, and a case series in MS and NMOSD. Neurol Neuroimmunol Neuroinflamm 2018;5(3):e453.

45. Friedrichs B, Tiemann M, Salwender H, et al. The effects of rituximab treatment during pregnancy on a neonate. Haematologica 2006;91(10):1426–7.

46. Buckley LM, Bullaboy CA, Leichtman L, et al. Multiple congenital anomalies associated with weekly low-dose methotrexate treatment of the mother. Arthritis Rheum 1997;40(5):971–3.

47. Hyoun SC, Obican SG, Scialli AR. Teratogen update: methotrexate. Birth Defects Res A Clin Mol Teratol 2012;94(4):187–207.

48. Dawson AL, Riehle-Colarusso T, Reefhuis J, et al. National Birth Defects Prevention Study. Maternal exposure to methotrexate and birth defects: a population-based study. Am J Med Genet A 2014;164A(9):2212–6.

49. Sifontis NM, Coscia LA, Constantinescu S, et al. Pregnancy outcomes in solid organ transplant recipients with exposure to mycophenolate mofetil or sirolimus. Transplantation 2006;82(12):1698–702.

50. Perez-Aytes A, Ledo A, Boso V, et al. In utero exposure to mycophenolate mofetil: a characteristic phenotype? Am J Med Genet A 2008;146A(1):1–7.

51. Cassina M, Johnson DL, Robinson LK, et al. Pregnancy outcome in women exposed to leflunomide before or during pregnancy. Arthritis Rheum 2012; 64(7):2085–94.

Telemedicine in Obstetrics

Adina R. Kern-Goldberger, MD, MPH, Sindhu K. Srinivas, MD, MSCE*

KEYWORDS

- Telemedicine • Telehealth • Mobile health • Access to care • Rural health
- Health disparities

KEY POINTS

- Telemedicine is an important modality of care delivery in the twenty-first century and has many applications for the obstetric population.
- Existing research has shown the clinical efficacy and improved patient satisfaction of many telemedicine platforms in obstetrics.
- Telemedicine has the potential to reduce racial and geographic disparities in pregnancy care, but more research is necessary to inform best practices.
- Developing cost-effective telemedicine programs and establishing health care policy that standardizes insurance reimbursement are some of the most important steps toward scaling up telemedicine offerings for obstetric patients in the United States.

INTRODUCTION

Innovations in telecommunication have transformed the world with mobile phones, wireless Internet, videochatting, and countless apps to perform nearly every function imaginable. They have also created the potential for significant advances in medicine via improved technology and increased access. The US Department of Health and Human services estimated in 2016 that most health care institutions in the United States, including hospitals, use some form of telecommunication to provide health care.[1] Given the rapid proliferation of these technologies in medicine, research is essential to inform evidence-based best practices for clinicians and consumers.[2] Applications of telecommunication technologies can have especial import in the obstetric population, for whom timely and convenient access to specialty care is critical. This article examines the ways that telecommunication tools have been applied to improve obstetric care.

Department of Obstetrics & Gynecology, Maternal Child Health Research Center, University of Pennsylvania Perelman School of Medicine, Hospital of the University of Pennsylvania, 3400 Spruce Street, 2nd Floor Silverstein Building, Philadelphia, PA 19146, USA
* Corresponding author.
E-mail address: ssrinivas@pennmedicine.upenn.edu

Clin Perinatol 47 (2020) 743–757
https://doi.org/10.1016/j.clp.2020.08.007
0095-5108/20/© 2020 Elsevier Inc. All rights reserved.

TELEHEALTH AND TELEMEDICINE

Telehealth, defined as the exchange of patient information via telecommunications from one site to another in order to improve patient health, has become a critical adjunctive component to the health care system in the United States.[3] The application of telehealth for diagnostic and treatment services, known as telemedicine, has emerged as an effective means of extending specialty medical care to hospitals and clinics in need, and can be used as a tool to overcome access barriers to equitable, high-quality health care. Telemedicine involves harnessing technology to manage patients through remote interactions that include audio or video real-time communications as well as review of data and images. It has the unique potential to obviate logistical and economic burdens that long-distance travel for medical care places on both patients and providers and offers new and creative approaches to the management of many medical conditions.[4]

Telemedicine tools can be used to facilitate communication and consultation between individual physicians as well as between health care providers and patients. This ability encompasses everything from off-site imaging interpretation by radiology to email communications between practitioners and patients on a health care Web portal to remote monitoring devices for blood glucose or heart rhythm that transmit real-time data (**Fig. 1**). As physicians continue to apply telemedicine to their practices in increasing numbers, there are several important national trends that are likely to influence the growth of telemedicine in the United States. First, consumer technologies in the health care sphere (such as wearable monitors) continue to evolve, and this entices increasing financial capital for product development. Electronic medical record and clinical-decision support software also continue to develop, which will allow further integration of telemedicine capabilities. From a structural standpoint, health care culture is becoming increasingly consumer focused with emphasis on efficient

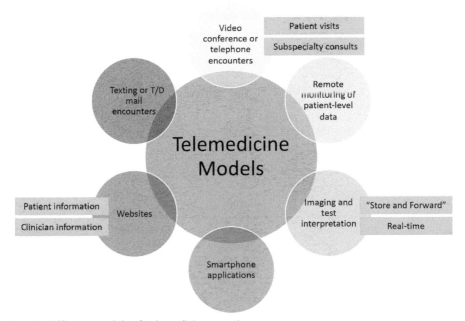

Fig. 1. Different models of telemedicine practice.

access to care and patient satisfaction, both of which can be enabled through tele-medicine. Further, significant physician shortages are projected in many fields in the coming years, which may require innovative telemedicine solutions.[3] Although the development and adoption of telemedicine technologies are subject to larger trends in health care economics and policy, all of these factors are likely to contribute to continued advancement in telemedicine. In addition, providing care via telemedicine may improve the practice of medicine by requiring providers to develop more advanced triage and history-taking skills, because fewer tools are available to them during remote evaluations. It may also promote more judicious use of medical testing and care escalation because the patients are not physically in front of the provider and any follow-up care may require the patients to physically relocate to a new facility.

Numerous health care fields have also successfully applied telemedicine platforms to acute and inpatient care. For instance, many hospitals are not adequately staffed by intensivists to provide needed coverage for critical care units, especially given increasing patient complexity and rapidly expanding medical technologies. Telemed-icine has been used for remote patient management in the intensive care unit and studies have shown similar and even improved patient outcomes, specifically with the outcomes of length of stay and mortality.[5,6] Telestroke care is another example of successful implementation of telemedicine technologies for acute patient manage-ment. Neurologists in these programs provide remote stroke consultations and can determine eligibility for thrombolytic administration, which has high time sensitivity, and data have shown decreased complications as well as lower in-hospital mortality.[7,8]

In obstetrics, telemedicine has emerged as an important tool to render outpatient care more convenient, pregnancy-complicating chronic diseases easier to manage, and subspecialty consult services and imaging more accessible. As telecommunica-tion technologies continue to advance rapidly and disparities in access to high-quality care continue to grow, telemedicine becomes an ever more critical element of peri-natal health care as a plausible solution to growing disparities. However, as telehealth strategies expand, implementation strategies need to ensure that disparities are not inadvertently widened.

PRENATAL AND POSTPARTUM CARE

A hallmark of routine obstetric care is regular prenatal visits with a physician or midwife to assess the pregnancy, provide education and counseling, and monitor for develop-ment of complications, with 13 to 14 total visits in a typical pregnancy.[9] A typical visit involves maternal vital signs, ascertainment of the fetal heart rate, assessment of uter-ine fundal height, and a urine dipstick at a minimum, with additional care based on the patient's gestational age and the presence of any comorbidities or developing compli-cations. For many low-risk patients, these visits may seem burdensome and disrup-tive, requiring time off from work, a commute to the provider's office, and a potential long wait to be evaluated for a short appointment, without uncovering a great deal of new information about the developing pregnancy. However, telemedicine can offer virtual prenatal care at the patient's convenience. Although not a complete replacement for in-person visits, telemedicine affords the opportunity for appropriate patients to obtain some of their care in a more convenient, patient-centered way.

One such program developed at the Mayo Clinic, called OB Nest, is a new model of care for low-risk pregnant women involving self-monitoring tools, a texting platform with the medical team, and an online community of other pregnant patients to share experiences.[10] Patients were provided with home kits including a blood pressure cuff, a hand-held Doppler, and urine dipsticks with instructions on how to perform these at home at regular intervals. Participating patients reported in interviews that obtaining their own measurements in the convenience and comfort of their own homes afforded them an increased sense of control, confidence, and reassurance during the pregnancy. Another innovative telemedicine-based prenatal care platform combined traditional in-person physician appointments with teleconference appointments and found no difference in obstetric outcomes compared with a completely traditional model.[11] Prenatal care programs such as these may be optimal for women who are not just low risk but also multiparous, and therefore require less in-person anticipatory guidance for pregnancy. A systematic review of 19 studies of telemedicine applications in low-risk obstetrics that each targeted specific elements of prenatal care (17 randomized controlled trials, 1 case-control study, 1 retrospective cohort) found variable success.[12] Smoking cessation interventions uniformly resulted in improved self-reported rates of smoking compared with usual care, and breastfeeding support programs were similarly successful. However, telemedicine programs to encourage vaccination for influenza did not show significant improvement from controls.

A growing body of research and health policy work in recent years has focused on the postpartum period, or fourth trimester, recognizing that this is a time of high medical and psychosocial risk for obstetric patients and that a large proportion of obstetric morbidity and mortality occurs during this time.[13] Postpartum care can similarly be retooled into telemedicine platforms to increase access, especially given historically poor rates of postpartum outpatient follow-up in general, and specifically in the highest-risk patient populations.[14] Telemedicine-mediated postpartum care may be particularly useful for screening and treatment of postpartum depression, for which diagnosis and treatment remain particularly challenging.[15] However, interventions such as telephone-based cognitive behavior therapy for perinatal depression are new, and further research is needed to assess feasibility and outcomes.[16,17] Telemedicine platforms for other specific aspects of perinatal care have been studied, including weight management and physical activity, with evidence of efficacy specifically in the postpartum period.[18,19] Research from other developed countries, including Sweden and Japan, has shown patient and provider satisfaction with telephone and videoconference-based consultations in the postpartum period to facilitate early hospital discharge and to support new mothers in the home setting.[20-22]

FETAL MONITORING

Telemedicine has also been used for remote fetal heart rate monitoring, both in the home setting as well as in the office of local providers. Cardiotocography, the standard of care for fetal heart rate monitoring, records the fetal heart rate using abdominal Doppler ultrasonography technology and is typically performed in hospital antenatal testing units or designated outpatient centers for women in the third trimester of pregnancy who require additional pregnancy surveillance with nonstress tests. This additional testing can be extremely inconvenient for patients, who must be absent from work or other family responsibilities 1 to 3 times per week depending on the frequency of testing. For women in more remote areas, a lengthy commute to an antenatal testing facility may also be involved. Telemedicine fetal monitoring could facilitate antenatal surveillance from the privacy, comfort, and convenience of patients' homes or a local provider's office. An Italian study investigating the performance of TOCO-MAT, a system for computerized antepartum cardiotocography and interpretation, at 9 peripheral sites found that decentralization of monitoring to remote sites facilitated increased access to care and improved patient quality of life.[23] Numerous additional studies evaluating other modalities of remote fetal heart rate monitoring, including phonocardiography and electrocardiography, showed acceptability, feasibility, reliability, and cost-effectiveness.[24–26] As with telemedicine-mediated prenatal care, remote fetal monitoring has the potential to empower patients by accommodating better to their lifestyles and bringing the care into their spaces. In addition, the innovative infant monitoring company Owlet is currently beta testing a direct-to-consumer fetal monitoring band that is purported to assess contractions and fetal heart rate, although is not credentialed or marketed as a medical device.[27]

Although there are potential improvements in comfort and convenience, telemedicine-based fetal monitoring could also incur certain risks. In the event of an abnormal result, which, in the case of fetal cardiotocography, could potentially require an emergent delivery, there is no capability for rapid, on-site medical intervention. The judiciousness of using a medical test under conditions that do not allow appropriate responsiveness when necessary should be carefully evaluated when considering implementing a remote fetal monitoring program. In addition, it is also possible that increased accessibility can promote medically unwarranted overuse of care. In traditional medical systems, the hassle of presenting for care exerts a natural force of checks and balances that, at least to some degree, prevents unnecessary evaluations, which is nullified by the utility of telemedicine. Overuse of care can in turn lead to an increase in false-positives, which can create a cascade of further unnecessary interventions. As an example, this has been addressed specifically with regard to home pulse oximeter monitors marketed to parents of infants, with concern for lack of accuracy and unintended consequences, including further unnecessary medical intervention.[28]

ULTRASONOGRAPHY, FETAL ECHOCARDIOGRAPHY, AND GENETICS

Obstetric ultrasonography is the key diagnostic tool for evaluating a developing pregnancy, including assessments of fetal viability and plurality, markers for aneuploidy, fetal anomalies, and fetal well-being. However, skilled ultrasonography interpretation is not readily available at many sites of obstetric clinical care. Telemedicine has the capability of allowing a scan performed by a sonographer in one location to be interpreted, either via a store-and-forward function or in real time, by an obstetrician or radiologist at another. Research as early as the 1990s showed the feasibility and accuracy of real-time teleultrasonography for the remote diagnosis of fetal structural anomalies.[29–31] Specifically, an early Australian study of teleultrasonography from this period showed that the original sonographic diagnosis was changed in 45.8% of cases when an ultrasonography scan was reinterpreted by an expert via a telemedicine program, and this led to 33.3% of cases necessitating a change in management.[32] Although technology has advanced since these studies were performed, facilitating easier remote ultrasonography interpretation with improved image quality because of the ability to transmit images over the Internet rather than through telephone lines, the principle of improved diagnostic accuracy when ultrasonography scans are read by experts holds just as true. More recent data from a large study of a teleultrasonography program in Arkansas, which used both store-and-forward still images and cine clips as well as real-time transmission with high-definition video, showed similar sensitivity and accuracy of teleultrasonography as published rates of on-site ultrasonography.[33] A validation study comparing the same teleultrasonography program with on-site ultrasonography found that teleultrasonography had inferior sensitivity compared with on-site ultrasonography but had higher accuracy as well as both positive and negative predictive values for detection of fetal anomalies.[34]

Another potential important application of telesonography is fetal echocardiography. Congenital cardiac defects are the most common birth defects in the United States,[35] and the ability to provide thorough antenatal diagnostic evaluation to allow prenatal counseling and management is critical. A large prospective study in the United Kingdom involved the performance of 3 fetal echocardiograms on each patient: the first by a sonographer alone, the second by a sonographer with real-time remote guidance by a pediatric cardiologist, and the third with a pediatric cardiologist on site. Findings included that the telemedicine-facilitated fetal echocardiogram was 97% accurate in diagnosing congenital heart disease compared with the gold standard of an in-person cardiologist. When surveyed, the sonographers in the study reported increased confidence and proficiency when they received real-time telemedicine support.[36] Other studies assessing technical feasibility of virtual fetal cardiac sonography from stored images using both three-dimensional and four-dimensional imaging have yielded promising results in terms of success in obtaining the necessary images, as well as accuracy and reliability.[37,38] Another study of telecardiology in Ireland found that participants preferred local telemedicine-mediated fetal echocardiography to face-to-face consultation at a regional medical center.[36]

Coupled with sonography, genetics counseling is an important aspect of prenatal care, including carrier screening, aneuploidy screening and diagnosis, and work-up of congenital anomalies. However, genetics providers both geneticists and genetic counselors, typically work in major academic centers and may not be readily accessible to patients in remote and rural areas. Patient satisfaction with telegenetic consultation in general has been well documented, although qualitative studies of practitioners have shown provider concern about their ability to establish rapport with patients via telecommunication.[39,40] Because prenatal genetics consultations can be highly sensitive and potentially involve difficult information and poor prognostication, it is especially important to ensure a therapeutic relationship between patient and provider to facilitate these conversations. More research is needed to assess the patient experience in the setting of prenatal telegenetics specifically, but a small qualitative study in Arkansas showed positive patient views of their experiences receiving difficult perinatal diagnoses via telemedicine.[41]

MATERNAL-FETAL MEDICINE CONSULTATION

The United States currently faces an epidemic of maternal morbidity and mortality, and gaps in maternal care are particularly glaring when maternal-fetal medicine (MFM) services are required but unavailable. MFM subspecialists, with advanced obstetric training focused on the management of high-risk pregnancies, play essential roles in many health systems, both in terms of direct patient care and clinical leadership.[42] Research has shown that the density of MFM specialists is inversely associated with maternal mortality and that MFM care during pregnancy is associated with later gestational age at delivery and shorter antepartum admissions.[43,44] Because maternal morbidity and mortality continue to be threats, MFM services are becoming increasingly vital and in demand.[42] However, there is a general shortage of MFM subspecialists to provide essential consultative, comanagement, and primary obstetric care for high-risk pregnant patients that may exacerbate the maternal morbidity and mortality crisis. MFM physicians tend to be concentrated in northeastern metropolitan areas and to practice in academic settings, rendering many areas of the country and many community-based obstetric hospitals uncovered.[45,46] Approximately 25 million reproductive-aged women live in counties without an available MFM subspecialist.[47]

Successful Models

Several states with large rural populations have established large telemedicine-based MFM programs (representative examples are shown in **Fig. 2**). The High Risk Pregnancy Program (formerly known as the Antenatal and Neonatal Guidelines, Education, and Learning System [ANGELS]) based at the University of Arkansas for Medical Sciences is the longest standing of these, established in 2002 to address the issue of access to MFM care in much of the state. ANGELS facilitates weekly telemedicine conferences between generalists and MFM subspecialists and provides real-time, telemedicine-based antenatal care, ultrasonography interpretation, telephone consultative support, and triage and transport services.[48,49] Solutions to Obstetrics in Rural Counties, a similar program that was developed in Tennessee, involves full-time telemedicine access to an MFM consultant for all rural hospitals in addition to an advanced practice provider and sonographer who make weekly in-person visits. Research has shown a high level of patient satisfaction from participation in the telemedicine program.[50] An observational study of a large telemedicine MFM program based in Pittsburgh comparing patients receiving telemedicine-based care with in-person care showed similar obstetric outcomes with cost savings of $90.28 per patient per consult as well as high patient satisfaction scores.[51]

Diabetes and Other Chronic Conditions

Diabetes care in pregnancy is a common application of maternal-fetal telemedicine. A pervasive feature of many diabetes programs in pregnancy is remote review of patient blood glucose logs, mediated through the glucometer itself or patient-initiated text messages or emails. This remote review allows providers to titrate treatment regimens regularly without necessitating additional in-person clinic visits, facilitating potentially improved compliance as well as diabetes-related pregnancy outcomes. Prior studies have shown at worst noninferiority and at best reduced rates of macrosomia and cesarean delivery in patients managed with telemedicine compared with controls seen more frequently in clinic for diabetes care.[52,53] A randomized trial of a smartphone-based daily prompt for diabetes care found higher rates of medication compliance, lower mean blood glucose levels, and lower rates of requiring insulin therapy compared with routine care.[54] A meta-analysis of telediabetes programs showed

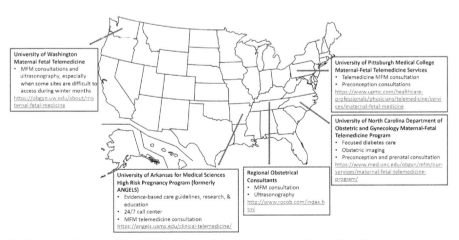

Fig. 2. Examples of existing MFM telemedicine programs in the United States.

comparable glycemic control, birth weight, and rates of cesarean delivery and neonatal intensive care admission with women who underwent traditional management. As rates of diabetes continue to increase in the setting of the obesity epidemic, thereby limiting traditional health care resources for these patients, telediabetes management technologies are rendered ever more crucial. Direct-to-consumer patient mobile applications for diabetes management have also rapidly proliferated in recent years, now numbering in the hundreds.[55] Progress has also been made in the realm of telemedicine-based asthma management in pregnancy. A randomized controlled trial investigating the use of a Bluetooth-enabled spirometer and an asthma mobile phone application in pregnant women found significant improvement in asthma symptoms after 6 months, compared with patients with traditional care.[56] There is ample potential for additional telemedicine platforms to assist in the management of other chronic conditions, such as hypertension, autoimmune disease, and heart disease, with features such as remote blood pressure monitoring and symptoms tracking.

Inpatient Management

Although existing paradigms have shown that maternal care for high-risk women is optimized through delivery at hospitals that can provide a broad array of subspecialty services as well as at hospitals with higher delivery volume,[57–59] the reality is that most women obtain care in hospitals and birth centers that provide only a basic level of care and perform fewer than 1000 deliveries per year.[60] These centers are of extreme practical importance, because they provide local health services for women in rural and often underserved communities.[61] However, when unanticipated obstetric acuity evolves, they may not be equipped to manage these situations without the guidance of MFM subspecialists or the availability of standardized response systems. Transferring patients to other hospitals can create a significant burden on families, especially when the nearest higher level of care is hundreds of kilometers away. In addition, and most importantly, transporting an actively decompensating patient is often not possible nor is it in the best interest of the patient. These realities necessitate the evaluation of a model where the subspecialty care is accessible at the bedside of every patient. Telemedicine has proved to be an extremely effective tool in managing acute and inpatient care in numerous nonobstetric settings as a surrogate for unavailable in-person subspecialty care.[62,63] At this point, telemedicine has not yet been applied in the inpatient obstetric context and it remains unknown whether MFM telemedicine management can improve outcomes in hospitals where in-person, inpatient MFM services are unavailable. Research is desperately needed in this area to evaluate the impact of MFM telemedicine management in the inpatient setting as a way to reduce maternal morbidity and mortality in hospitals with limited access to needed resources and care.

MOBILE PHONE TECHNOLOGIES

Mobile phone technologies open worlds of possibility for innovating obstetric care. Mobile health (also known as mHealth) exists in 2 primary modalities: texting-based programs and mobile phone applications. There is ample evidence of the success of mobile phone applications to support good health behaviors and to facilitate health care delivery in general.[64–66] In the past decade there has been rapid development in the market of direct-to-consumer women's health and pregnancy mobile applications, accounting for 7% of all apps in 2015.[67] The Text4baby program of the National Healthy Mothers Health Babies Coalition is a large health education initiative wherein women receive text messages with health information about the pregnancy and the baby through the first year of life.[68] Other text-based platforms have been developed for breastfeeding support, smoking cessation, vaccination, and physical wellness. The efficacy of these programs is mixed, with generally more success in interventions that support an ongoing behavior, such as breastfeeding or smoking cessation, as opposed to initiating a new behavior such as vaccination or increased physical activity.[12] Mobile phone telemedicine programs have also evolved specifically around the postpartum management of hypertensive disorders of pregnancy. In a randomized trial, text-based remote blood pressure monitoring in the postpartum period has been shown to be more effective at obtaining blood pressure readings than scheduling patients for office follow-up.[69] Studies assessing implementation parameters of these mobile phone platforms for postpartum hypertension have shown feasibility as well as patient satisfaction.[70,71]

TELEMEDICINE AND HEALTH DISPARITIES

Obstetric morbidity disproportionately affects women with difficult access to care, including those facing socioeconomic and geographic barriers, as well as women from minority racial and ethnic backgrounds.[72–74] Telemedicine, with its unique ability to connect patients to high-level care remotely, has the potential to alleviate this problem. Data from the ANGELS telemedicine program in Arkansas have shown that, among patients with Medicaid insurance, the rate of very-low-birth-weight infants delivered in hospitals without a neonatal intensive care unit decreased significantly,[75] which suggests a meaningful targeted improvement in perinatal care for women facing both socioeconomic and geographic challenges to care. A study of a text-message postpartum blood pressure monitoring program found that, compared with usual care, in which black women are only half as likely to obtain recommended hypertension follow-up, there was a 50% reduction in this disparity between black and nonblack women who participated in the telemedicine program.[76] However, low resources and poor health literacy can also predispose already disadvantaged women from participating successfully in telemedicine interventions, as seen in the Text4baby program, in which women were more likely to successfully enroll and participate if they had more education, higher income, and smaller household size.[77] Because compromised access to necessary medical services disproportionately affects women from minority racial and ethnic backgrounds as well as from rural areas, obstetric providers should continue to cultivate creative telemedicine strategies to effect better outcomes for these vulnerable populations.

HEALTH POLICY IMPLICATIONS

The adoption and scalability of any telemedicine program is ultimately subject to the politics of health insurance coverage. Reimbursement policies for telemedicine by Medicaid and commercial insurers are determined at the state level, whereas the federal government determines similar guidelines for Medicare.[78] The current, and very narrow, criteria for Medicare telemedicine reimbursement specify the provision of service to a rural Health Professional Shortage Area to patients with diabetes, end-stage renal disease, or psychiatric disease or for emergency department or skilled nursing facility care in specific specialties.[79] In contrast, state-level policies remain highly variable. Only 3 states (Ohio, North Carolina, New York) specifically discuss perinatal telemedicine, although 32 have laws requiring private insurers to reimburse telemedicine services at a comparable rate with in-person services.[80,81] However, there is significant variation in the realities of reimbursement for telemedicine even when it is covered, and many private insurers do not routinely reimburse for telemedicine services at all.[82] In order to implement truly large-scale, systematic telemedicine programs in obstetrics, as with any field, standardized insurance reimbursement is essential. Evidence of telemedicine's favorable medical outcomes, improved provider and patient satisfaction, and demonstrated cost-effectiveness should incentivize both state and federal policymakers to craft strategic reimbursement plans for telemedicine services that will enable these programs to expand effectively. These policies should specifically address the perinatal population and the importance of providing timely and risk-appropriate care so that telemedicine can be used as a platform to provide efficient care and effectively extend the necessary level of care to resource-poor communities.[80]

STRATEGIES FOR SUCCESSFUL TELEMEDICINE IMPLEMENTATION IN OBSTETRICS

A successful telemedicine program addresses the values of all relevant stakeholders, including patients and families, health care systems, consulting and referring physicians, and payers, which may be different from priorities in traditional health care.[78] For patients, these programs should optimize convenience and ease of use in order to justify the lack of a traditional face-to-face encounter with a physician that many patients expect. For physicians and health systems, telemedicine programs must have the ability to improve clinical outcomes by bringing care to underserved populations and must be able to provide the consulting physician with high-quality data in order to provide high-quality care. Telemedicine, by definition, depends on technology, and ensuring adequate and up-to-date technological capacity is critical for a successful telemedicine program. This capacity can involve cloud-based storage and transfer of images, video conferencing, computer and speaker systems, software, and mobile devices such as cellular phones and tablets. A framework has been designed to evaluate telemedicine programs, The Model for Assessment of Telemedicine Applications (MAST), and it recommends multidisciplinary assessment of several key components of every telemedicine program after implementation in order to achieve success: the health problem of interest; safety; clinical effectiveness; cost-effectiveness; patient perspectives; and sociocultural, legal, and ethical attributes.[83]

BARRIERS TO TELEMEDICINE IN OBSTETRICS

Although telemedicine offers an innovative solution to the problem of access to care and potentially to the larger issue of obstetric morbidity and mortality, it also faces numerous barriers to widespread uptake. The primary barrier is standardized insurance reimbursement, as already discussed.[84] Additional challenges include state-based licensure and credentialing systems, which could render it difficult for physicians to provide telemedicine services across state lines, and malpractice liability, because there is not yet a standardized model for telemedicine.[85] There are also unique concerns related to data security, given that telemedicine inherently involves the transmission of health information. Cost is also a potential significant barrier to telemedicine success. One of the specific issues complicating cost-effectiveness for telemedicine-based consultative services is the need to reimburse both the referring site as well as the consult, and there is no established model at present to accomplish this. Existing studies on the cost-effectiveness of obstetric telemedicine have been small, and it can be challenging to quantify some of the benefits of telemedicine, such as reduced travel time.[86]

SUMMARY

Obstetric telemedicine is reshaping the way that perinatal health care is provided, from restructuring outpatient prenatal care and postpartum follow-up to extending advanced imaging such as fetal anatomy sonography and echocardiography to rural areas, and it continues to evolve rapidly concomitant with the technological advances of the twenty-first century. More research is necessary to further clarify best practices for the many variegated applications of telemedicine in pregnancy care and specifically focus on reducing health disparities and optimizing cost-effectiveness. Recent world events have shown that having a functional and scalable telemedicine infrastructure that can be operationalized in times of pandemic or other national emergencies is critical to ensure the ongoing, safe, and successful practice of medicine.

CLINICS CARE POINTS

- Providing obstetric care via telemedicine can increase access while maintaining high-quality.
- Obstetric telemedicine programs should account for cost and appropriate infrastructure to ensure effective implementation and sustainability.
- Telemedicine in obstetrics has the potential to reduce barriers and disparities but could also widen inequalities if not operationalized successfully.

DISCLOSURE

The authors report no conflict of interest.

REFERENCES

1. Report to congress: E-health and tele-medicine. Department of Health and Human Services, Office of Health Policy, Office of the Assistant Secretary for Planning and Evaluation; 2016.
2. Totten AM, Womack DM, Eden KB, et al. In: Telehealth: mapping the evidence for patient outcomes from systematic reviews. Rockville (MD): Agency for Healthcare Research; 2016.
3. Tuckson RV, Edmunds M, Hodgkins ML. Telehealth. N Engl J Med 2017;377(16): 1585–92.
4. Field MJ, editor. Telemedicine: a guide to assessing telecommunications in health care. Washington, DC: National Academic Press; 1996.
5. Thomas EJ, Lucke JF, Wueste L, et al. Association of telemedicine for remote monitoring of intensive care patients with mortality, complications, and length of stay. JAMA 2009;302(24):2671–8.
6. Udeh C, Udeh B, Rahman N, et al. Telemedicine/virtual ICU: where are we and where are we going? Methodist Debakey Cardiovasc J 2018;14(2):126–33.
7. Wechsler LR, Demaerschalk BM, Schwamm LH, et al. Telemedicine quality and outcomes in stroke: a scientific statement for healthcare professionals from the American Heart Association/American Stroke Association. Stroke 2017;48(1): e3–25.
8. Zhang D, Shi L, Ido MS, et al. Impact of participation in a Telestroke network on clinical outcomes. Circ Cardiovasc Qual Outcomes 2019;12(1):e005147.
9. American Academy of Pediatrics TACoOG. Guidelines for perinatal care. 8th edition 2017.
10. de Mooij MJM, Hodny RL, O'Neil DA, et al. OB nest: reimagining low-risk prenatal care. Mayo Clin Proc 2018;93(4):458–66.

11. Pflugeisen BM, McCarren C, Poore S, et al. Virtual visits: managing prenatal care with modern technology. MCN Am J Matern Child Nurs 2016;41(1):24–30.

12. DeNicola N, Grossman D, Marko K, et al. Telehealth interventions to improve obstetric and gynecologic health outcomes: a systematic review. Obstet Gynecol 2020;135(2):371–82.

13. Callaghan WM, Creanga AA, Kuklina EV. Severe maternal morbidity among delivery and postpartum hospitalizations in the United States. Obstet Gynecol 2012; 120(5):1029–36.

14. Levine LD, Nkonde-Price C, Limaye M, et al. Factors associated with postpartum follow-up and persistent hypertension among women with severe preeclampsia. J Perinatol 2016;36(12):1079–82.

15. Learman LA. Screening for depression in pregnancy and the postpartum period. Clin Obstet Gynecol 2018;61(3):525–32.

16. Logsdon MC, Foltz MP, Stein B, et al. Adapting and testing telephone-based depression care management intervention for adolescent mothers. Arch Womens Ment Health 2010;13(4):307–17.

17. Nair U, Armfield NR, Chatfield MD, et al. The effectiveness of telemedicine interventions to address maternal depression: a systematic review and meta-analysis. J Telemed Telecare 2018;24(10):639–50.

18. Sherifali D, Nerenberg KA, Wilson S, et al. The effectiveness of eHealth technologies on weight management in pregnant and postpartum women: systematic review and meta-analysis. J Med Internet Res 2017;19(10):e337.

19. Fjeldsoe BS, Miller YD, Marshall AL. MobileMums: a randomized controlled trial of an SMS-based physical activity intervention. Ann Behav Med 2010;39(2):101–11.

20. Lindberg I, Ohrling K, Christensson K. Midwives' experience of using videoconferencing to support parents who were discharged early after childbirth. J Telemed Telecare 2007;13:202–5.

21. Lindberg I, Christensson K, Ohrling K. Parents' experiences of using videoconferencing as a support in early discharge after childbirth. Midwifery 2009;25: 357–65.

22. Kobayashi H, Sado T. Satisfaction of a new telephone consultation service for prenatal and postnatal health care. J Obstet Gynaecol Res 2019;45(7):1376–81.

23. Di Lieto A, De Falco M, Campanile M, et al. Regional and international prenatal telemedicine network for computerized antepartum cardiotocography. Telemed J E Health 2008;14(1):49–54.

24. Kovacs F, Torok M, Horvath C, et al. A new, phonocardiography-based telemetric fetal home monitoring system. Telemed J E Health 2010;16(8):878–82.

25. Rauf Z, O'Brien E, Stampalija T, et al. Home labour induction with retrievable prostaglandin pessary and continuous telemetric trans-abdominal fetal ECG monitoring. PLoS One 2011;6(11):e28129.

26. Schramm K, Lapert F, Nees J, et al. Acceptance of a new non-invasive fetal monitoring system and attitude for telemedicine approaches in obstetrics: a case-control study. Arch Gynecol Obstet 2018;298(6):1085–93.

27. Merrell C. Owlet announces its newest innovation: the owlet band, a prenatal wellness product. Owlet. 2019. Available at: https://blog.owletcare.com/owlet-announces-its-newest-innovation-the-owlet-band-a-prenatal-wellness-product/. Accessed March 2, 2020.

28. Bonafide CP, Localio AR, Ferro DF, et al. Accuracy of pulse oximetry-based home baby monitors. JAMA 2018;320(7):717–9.

29. Landwehr JB Jr, Zador IE, Wolfe HM, et al. Telemedicine and fetal ultrasonography: assessment of technical performance and clinical feasibility. Am J Obstet Gynecol 1997;177(4):846–8.
30. Fisk NM, Sepulveda W, Drysdale K, et al. Fetal telemedicine: six month pilot of real-time ultrasound and video consultation between the Isle of Wight and London. Br J Obstet Gynaecol 1996;103(11):1092–5.
31. Chan FY, Soong B, Watson D, et al. Realtime fetal ultrasound by telemedicine in Queensland. A successful venture? J Telemed Telecare 2001;7(Suppl 2):7–11.
32. Chan FY, Soong B, Lessing K, et al. Clinical value of real-time tertiary fetal ultrasound consultation by telemedicine: preliminary evaluation. Telemed J 2000;6(2):237–42.
33. Rabie NZ, Sandlin AT, Barber KA, et al. Teleultrasound: how accurate are we? J Ultrasound Med 2017;36(11):2329–35.
34. Rabie NZ, Sandlin AT, Ounpraseuth S, et al. Teleultrasound for pre-natal diagnosis: a validation study. AJUM 2019;22(4).
35. Hoffman JI, Kaplan S. The incidence of congenital heart disease. J Am Coll Cardiol 2002;39(12):1890–900.
36. McCrossan BA, Sands AJ, Kileen T, et al. Fetal diagnosis of congenital heart disease by telemedicine. Arch Dis Child Fetal Neonatal Ed 2011;96(6):F394–7.
37. Espinoza J, Lee W, Comstock C, et al. Collaborative study on 4-dimensional echocardiography for the diagnosis of fetal heart defects: the COFEHD study. J Ultrasound Med 2010;29(11):1573–80.
38. Michailidis GD, Simpson JM, Karidas C, et al. Detailed three-dimensional fetal echocardiography facilitated by an Internet link. Ultrasound Obstet Gynecol 2001;18(4):325–8.
39. Zilliacus EM, Meiser B, Lobb EA, et al. Women's experience of telehealth cancer genetic counseling. J Genet Couns 2010;19(5):463–72.
40. Hilgart JS, Hayward JA, Coles B, et al. Telegenetics: a systematic review of telemedicine in genetics services. Genet Med 2012;14(9):765–76.
41. Wyatt SN, Rhoads SJ, Green AL, et al. Maternal response to high-risk obstetric telemedicine consults when perinatal prognosis is poor. Aust N Z J Obstet Gynaecol 2013;53(5):494–7.
42. Society for Maternal-Fetal M, Sciscione A, Berghella V, et al. Society for maternal-fetal medicine (SMFM) special report: the maternal-fetal medicine subspecialists' role within a health care system. Am J Obstet Gynecol 2014;211(6):607–16.
43. Sullivan SA, Hill EG, Newman RB, et al. Maternal-fetal medicine specialist density is inversely associated with maternal mortality ratios. Am J Obstet Gynecol 2005;193(3 Pt 2):1083–8.
44. Eden RD, Penka A, Britt DW, et al. Re-evaluating the role of the MFM specialist: lead, follow, or get out of the way. J Matern Fetal Neonatal Med 2005;18(4):253–8.
45. Sisson MC, Witcher PM, Stubsten C. The role of the maternal-fetal medicine specialist in high-risk obstetric care. Crit Care Nurs Clin North Am 2004;16(2):187–91.
46. Pearse WH, Gant NF, Hagner AP. Workforce projections for subspecialists in obstetrics and gynecology. Obstet Gynecol 2000;95(2):312–4.
47. D'Alton ME, Friedman AM, Bernstein PS, et al. Putting the "M" back in maternal-fetal medicine: a 5-year report card on a collaborative effort to address maternal morbidity and mortality in the United States. Am J Obstet Gynecol 2019;221(4):311–7.e1.

48. Britt DW, Norton JD, Lowery CL. Equity in the development of telemedicine sites in an Arkansas high-risk pregnancy programme. J Telemed Telecare 2006;12(5): 242–5.

49. Lowery C, Bronstein J, McGhee J, et al. ANGELS and University of Arkansas for Medical Sciences paradigm for distant obstetrical care delivery. Am J Obstet Gynecol 2007;196(6):534.e1-9.

50. Wood D. STORC helps deliver healthy babies: the telemedicine program that serves rural women with high-risk pregnancies. Telemed J E Health 2011; 17(1):2–4.

51. Leighton C, Conroy M, Bilderback A, et al. Implementation and impact of a maternal-fetal medicine telemedicine program. Am J Perinatol 2019;36(7):751–8.

52. Ladyzynski P, Wojcicki JM, Krzymien J, et al. Teletransmission system supporting intensive insulin treatment of out-clinic type 1 diabetic pregnant women. Technical assessment during 3 years' application. Int J Artif Organs 2001;24(3): 157–63.

53. Perez-Ferre N, Galindo M, Fernandez MD, et al. The outcomes of gestational diabetes mellitus after a telecare approach are not inferior to traditional outpatient clinic visits. Int J Endocrinol 2010;2010:386941.

54. Miremberg H, Ben-Ari T, Betzer T, et al. The impact of a daily smartphone-based feedback system among women with gestational diabetes on compliance, glycemic control, satisfaction, and pregnancy outcome: a randomized controlled trial. Am J Obstet Gynecol 2018;218(4):453.e1-7.

55. Chomutare T, Fernandez-Luque L, Arsand E, et al. Features of mobile diabetes applications: review of the literature and analysis of current applications compared against evidence-based guidelines. J Med Internet Res 2011; 13(3):e65.

56. Zairina E, Abramson MJ, McDonald CF, et al. Telehealth to improve asthma control in pregnancy: a randomized controlled trial. Respirology 2016;21(5):867–74.

57. Ananth CV, Lavery JA, Friedman AM, et al. Serious maternal complications in relation to severe pre-eclampsia: a retrospective cohort study of the impact of hospital volume. BJOG 2017;124(8):1246–53.

58. Janakiraman V, Lazar J, Joynt KE, et al. Hospital volume, provider volume, and complications after childbirth in U.S. hospitals. Obstet Gynecol 2011;118(3): 521–7.

59. Wright JD, Herzog TJ, Shah M, et al. Regionalization of care for obstetric hemorrhage and its effect on maternal mortality. Obstet Gynecol 2010;115(6):1194–200.

60. Simpson KR. An overview of distribution of births in United States hospitals in 2008 with implications for small volume perinatal units in rural hospitals. J Obstet Gynecol Neonatal Nurs 2011;40(4):432–9.

61. Levels of maternal care: obstetric care consensus No, 9. Obstet Gynecol 2019; 134(2):e41–55.

62. Flodgren G, Rachas A, Farmer AJ, et al. Interactive telemedicine: effects on professional practice and health care outcomes. Cochrane Database Syst Rev 2015;(9):CD002098.

63. Dorsey ER, Topol EJ. State of telehealth. N Engl J Med 2016;375(14):1400.

64. Cole-Lewis H, Kershaw T. Text messaging as a tool for behavior change in disease prevention and management. Epidemiol Rev 2010;32:56–69.

65. Fjeldsoe BS, Marshall AL, Miller YD. Behavior change interventions delivered by mobile telephone short-message service. Am J Prev Med 2009;36(2):165–73.

66. Whittaker R, McRobbie H, Bullen C, et al. Mobile phone-based interventions for smoking cessation. Cochrane Database Syst Rev 2016;4:CD006611.

67. Aitken M. Patient adoption of mHealth: use, evidence and remaining barriers to mainstream acceptance. IMS Institute for Healthcare Informatics; 2015.
68. Whittaker R, Matoff-Stepp S, Meehan J, et al. Text4baby: development and implementation of a national text messaging health information service. Am J Public Health 2012;102(12):2207–13.
69. Hirshberg A, Downes K, Srinivas S. Comparing standard office-based follow-up with text-based remote monitoring in the management of postpartum hypertension: a randomised clinical trial. BMJ Qual Saf 2018;27(11):871–7.
70. Rhoads SJ, Serrano CI, Lynch CE, et al. Exploring implementation of m-health monitoring in postpartum women with hypertension. Telemed J E Health 2017; 23(10):833–41.
71. Hoppe KK, Williams M, Thomas N, et al. Telehealth with remote blood pressure monitoring for postpartum hypertension: a prospective single-cohort feasibility study. Pregnancy Hypertens 2019;15:171–6.
72. Creanga AA, Bateman BT, Kuklina EV, et al. Racial and ethnic disparities in severe maternal morbidity: a multistate analysis, 2008-2010. Am J Obstet Gynecol 2014;210(5):435.e1-8.
73. Louis JM, Menard MK, Gee RE. Racial and ethnic disparities in maternal morbidity and mortality. Obstet Gynecol 2015;125(3):690–4.
74. ACOG Committee Opinion No. 429: health disparities for rural women. Obstet Gynecol 2009;113(3):762–5.
75. Kim EW, Teague-Ross TJ, Greenfield WW, et al. Telemedicine collaboration improves perinatal regionalization and lowers statewide infant mortality. J Perinatol 2013;33(9):725–30.
76. Hirshberg A, Sammel MD, Srinivas SK. Text message remote monitoring reduced racial disparities in postpartum blood pressure ascertainment. Am J Obstet Gynecol 2019;221(3):283–5.
77. Gazmararian JA, Elon L, Yang B, et al. Text4baby program: an opportunity to reach underserved pregnant and postpartum women? Matern Child Health J 2014;18(1):223–32.
78. Greiner AL. Telemedicine applications in obstetrics and gynecology. Clin Obstet Gynecol 2017;60(4):853–66.
79. Telehealth services. Center for Medicare and Medicaid Services; 2015.
80. Okoroh EM, Kroelinger CD, Smith AM, et al. US and territory telemedicine policies: identifying gaps in perinatal care. Am J Obstet Gynecol 2016;215(6): 772.e1-6.
81. Yang Y. Health policy brief: telehealth parity laws. Bethesda (MD): Health Affairs; 2016.
82. Asch DA. The hidden economics of telemedicine. Ann Intern Med 2015;163(10): 801–2.
83. Kidholm K, Ekeland AG, Jensen LK, et al. A model for assessment of telemedicine applications: mast. Int J Technol Assess Health Care 2012;28(1):44–51.
84. NCSL Partnership Project on Telehealth. Telehealth Policy Trends and Considerations. USA: National Conference of State Legislatures.
85. Odibo IN, Wendel PJ, Magann EF. Telemedicine in obstetrics. Clin Obstet Gynecol 2013;56(3):422–33.
86. Magann EF, McKelvey SS, Hitt WC, et al. The use of telemedicine in obstetrics: a review of the literature. Obstet Gynecol Surv 2011;66(3):170–8.

Clinical Implications of Maternal Disparities Administrative Data Research

Alexander Friedman, MD

KEYWORDS

- Maternal disparities • Maternal outcomes • Maternal safety
- Severe maternal morbidity

KEY POINTS

- Failure to rescue is likely an important contributor to maternal disparities.
- Risk for individual adverse outcomes by maternal race is differential.
- Optimal longitudinal care utilization with nonobstetric specialists is required to mitigate risk.

INTRODUCTION

Racial disparities in maternal outcomes are a major public health problem in the United States. The disproportionately high maternal mortality rate of non-Hispanic black women accounts for a significant proportion of the differential between the maternal mortality rate in the United States and other wealthy countries with lower maternal mortality rates. Data from the Centers for Disease Control and Prevention's Pregnancy Mortality Surveillance System demonstrated that risk for mortality is highest among non-Hispanic black women with a 3.4 mortality ratio for non-Hispanic black compared with non-Hispanic white women.[1,2] Increased risk for severe morbidity among non-Hispanic black women has been demonstrated across a broad range of clinical outcomes.[3–6] Although large outcome differentials by maternal race have been noted for non-Hispanic black women, there are major knowledge gaps related to the causes and mechanisms by which these disparities occur.

In seeking to reduce disparities, clinicians may consult maternal outcomes research. An important consideration in clinical interpretation of maternal outcomes disparities research is that analyses often use administrative data. Although

Conflicts of Interest: none.
Division of Maternal-Fetal Fetal Medicine, Department of Obstetrics and Gynecology, College of Physicians and Surgeons, Columbia University, 622 West 168th Street, PH 16-66, New York, NY 10032, USA
E-mail address: alexander.friedman@gmail.com

Clin Perinatol 47 (2020) 759–767
https://doi.org/10.1016/j.clp.2020.08.008

administrative data have many advantages including that it is readily available and appropriate for evaluating disease burden and resource utilization in large populations, it also has significant shortcomings that limit what causal inferences may be reasonably made.[7,8] Given the public health importance of maternal disparities, the purpose of this study is to review research with commonly used administrative data to identify major knowledge gaps and determine what inferences can be drawn regarding how maternal care can be improved to reduce disparities.

This review has 3 sections. First, the structures of commonly used administrative databases will be reviewed focusing on the National (Nationwide) Inpatient Sample (NIS). Second, administrative data maternal disparities research will be reviewed. Third, opportunities for improving clinical care and reducing disparities supported by inferences from administrative data research will be explored.

OVERVIEW OF ADMINISTRATIVE DATA RESEARCH

In determining which type of data to use for an analysis, a researcher may have several options including administrative data (which are often compiled for billing or vital statistics purposes), data from large multicenter studies, single-center research data, and data from the electronic health record. Different sources of data have varying advantages and disadvantages. Advantages of administrative data include that it may be population-level and able to facilitate good-quality population estimates, that it includes large number of rare outcomes, that it is readily available, and that very often linkages are available to other data sources for factors such as cost, detailed hospital characteristics, and other factors.[9] Given these strengths, administrative data are often used in maternal disparities outcomes research because it allows for statistically meaningful comparisons of relatively rare outcomes between different racial and ethnic groups. Major disadvantages, which will be subsequently explored, include that secondary diagnoses may or may not be well coded (as the primary purpose of administrative data is often billing) and misclassification can occur wherein preexisting conditions are coded as acute and vice versa.

Administrative data may come in several different formats that determine which factors can be analyzed. Many of the most commonly used databases such as those provided by the Healthcare Cost and Utilization Project sponsored by the Agency for Healthcare Research and Quality including the NIS, the Nationwide Readmissions Database (NRD), and the State Inpatient Databases include hospital discharge information including diagnosis codes, demographics, hospital characteristics, and charges.[10] For databases such as the NRD, patients can be followed-up over time within a state within a given year such that readmissions or other subsequent hospitalizations can be identified. For the NIS and NRD and similar databases, detailed information about clinical management during the hospitalization beyond billing codes are otherwise not available. Outpatient management is likewise not available. Other administrative databases may include more detailed information depending on the source of the data. In comparison to the NIS and NRD, a database such as Premier Perspective is composed of data contributed by hospitals.[11–14] Perspective includes hospitalization information such as drug and device administration allowing for more granular analysis of inpatient clinical management. Finally, payer databases may be a rich source of information related to health care utilization that includes outpatient services. Databases such as MarketScan include both commercial and Medicaid enrollees and can be used to follow patients through time capturing acute care hospitalizations, ambulatory care, emergency department utilization, pharmacy claims, and other health utilization.[15]

The National Inpatient Sample

The NIS from the Healthcare Cost and Utilization Project is a commonly used administrative database used to evaluate care and outcomes across specialties in the United States.[9] The database includes 20% of all hospitalizations from US community hospitals excluding rehabilitation and long-term acute care hospitals. At present, the data are included from 47 states plus the District of Columbia accounting for more than 97% of the US population, and the 20% of hospitalizations included can be weighted to provide full national estimates for the entire United States. A major advantage of this database is that given the large sample, rare conditions, uncommon treatments, and specific patient populations can be analyzed with numerators large enough to make meaningful statistical comparisons.

The NIS contains clinical and resource-use information typically found in hospital discharge abstracts. Clinical data are inferred from International Classification of Diseases, Ninth Revision, Clinical Modification (ICD-9-CM) diagnosis, procedure, and external cause of injury codes before the third quarter of 2015 and International Classification of Diseases, Tenth Revision, Clinical Modification (ICD-10-CM) diagnosis, procedures, and external cause of morbidity codes beginning from the fourth quarter of 2015 on. Other data include patient demographic characteristics (eg, sex, age, race, median household income for ZIP Code, payer), hospital characteristics (eg, ownership, region, rurality, teaching status), total hospital charges, discharge status, length of stay, and severity and comorbidity measures.[9] The NIS is frequently used for analyses related to health care utilization, inpatient care for rare conditions, variation in care, health care costs, national estimates of resource utilization, safety and quality of care, the impact of health policy, and access to care. In addition to the large populations included and the ability to create national estimates, the NIS has several advantages for researchers including that it is inexpensive to purchase, that the data files are relatively easy to use, and that 30 years of data (1988–2017) are currently available.

In evaluating obstetric outcomes in the NIS, the unit of analysis is often delivery hospitalizations although both antepartum and postpartum hospitalizations can be identified using billing codes specific to obstetric diagnoses. Maternal outcome studies in the NIS will often analyze a cohort of women hospitalized for delivery focusing on an outcome or set of outcomes and evaluating specific exposures. For example, maternal disparities analyses in the NIS might (1) identify women hospitalized for delivery; (2) further stratify the sample to evaluate a risk factor such as preeclampsia, postpartum hemorrhage, lupus, delivery at a black-serving hospital, or advanced maternal age[4,5,16,17]; and (3) determine the association between race and adverse outcomes in the finalized cross-sectional sample. Analyses with this type of research framework may provide a reasonable estimate of disease burden and the effect of race, provided that the exposures and outcomes are of reasonable validity. However, inferring causation from cross-sectional designs may be challenging based on significant limitations of the data, which include the following: (1) it is not always possible to determine whether a complication occurred before or during the hospital admission, (2) secondary billing diagnoses for chronic conditions may be poorly captured limiting case-mix adjustment, (3) secondary billing diagnoses for chronic conditions may not describe disease severity, (4) there may be no way of modeling longitudinal health care utilization such as prenatal care, and (5) there may be misclassification wherein conditions are not captured accurately.[7,18,19] All of these limitations may be of importance in considering how to translate research into clinical interventions that reduce maternal disparities.

MATERNAL DISPARITIES ADMINISTRATIVE DATA RESEARCH

Maternal administrative data research may provide important clinical insights helpful in reducing disparities. Three sets of findings are reviewed here: (1) there is a gradient with regard to severity of risk for non-Hispanic black women, (2) disparities in risk for individual adverse outcomes by race is differential, and (3) there are significant disparities in preventable adverse outcomes.

In conceptualizing maternal risk, it may be helpful to stratify women based on successive levels of risk for adverse outcomes. A broad finding in maternal disparities research is that although non-Hispanic black women are at modestly increased likelihood for common complications, they are at high risk for subsequent severe morbidity and even higher risk for death. For example, evaluating delivery hospitalizations in the NIS complicated by preeclampsia, overall risk for preeclampsia was modestly increased for non-Hispanic black women, but risks for severe morbidity such as stroke and acute renal failure were more than double that of non-Hispanic white women. In this study overall morbidity was 60% higher for black women and risk for death was 230% higher for non-Hispanic black women compared with other women.[4] Evaluating postpartum hemorrhage in the NIS, non-Hispanic black women were at similar risk for the condition but experienced large differentials in risk for overall severe morbidity, disseminated intravascular coagulation, transfusion, and hysterectomy compared with non-Hispanic white women.[5] Comparing non-Hispanic black women with other women with postpartum hemorrhage, non-Hispanic black women were at greater than 5 times the risk of death. A broad inference from these findings is that although non-Hispanic black women may be at modestly increased risk for common complications such as hypertension and hemorrhage based on underlying risk factors and comorbidity, clinical management and hospital factors are likely important contributors to the larger racial disparities in major adverse outcomes.

Another important insight of maternal disparities research is that risk for individual adverse outcomes by race is differential. For example, an NIS study of postpartum readmissions found that non-Hispanic black women were at significantly higher risk to be readmitted postpartum and to suffer severe maternal morbidity during readmission. They were at particularly high risk for pulmonary edema and acute heart failure, with these diagnoses present 126% more often than for non-Hispanic white women readmitted postpartum.[3] However, in evaluating risk for shock, hysterectomy, and disseminated intravascular coagulation, risk was lower for non-Hispanic black women or similar compared with non-Hispanic white women. In a different study evaluating obstetric venous thromboembolism (VTE) in the NIS the odds ratio for events among non-Hispanic black women was 1.4.[20] This estimate decreased from unadjusted models. Although a 40% increase in odds may seem to be a sizable differential, this risk is less than the magnitude at which population estimates with administrative data may be highly likely to identify true risk; it is important to consider that risk adjustment is likely incomplete and that once unmeasured confounding is accounted for there is a significant possibility that the effect of race will be nonsignificant. In addition, there are concerns about validity of obstetric VTE codes, and if misclassification occurs differentially by group estimates may not be valid.[19,21,22] These findings broadly demonstrate that risk differentials by race are not uniform and that robust models of risk will likely need to be cause specific as opposed to generalized. Given that there are no obstetric interventions that are likely to result in major increase or decrease in cardiac complication risk, a reasonable inference is that underlying comorbidity may affect risk.

Finally, maternal outcomes research supports that there may be "low-hanging fruit" in reducing disparities in that significant differentials are present in potentially avoidable adverse outcomes. Maternal stroke may be an important representative clinical example. On detailed review, most of the maternal deaths from stroke are preventable with better hypertension management.[23,24] Maternal stroke, comprising cerebral ischemic and infarction, subarachnoid hemorrhage (SAH), and intracerebral hemorrhage (ICH), complicates approximately 30 per 100,000 deliveries,[25] and up to 1 in 500 pregnancies is complicated by preeclampsia.[26] Up to 20% of maternal strokes are fatal,[25] and ICH is a leading cause of death in women with preeclampsia.[27–29] Most maternal strokes occur postpartum, often after women have been discharged home after delivery.[25] There are significant disparities in maternal stroke,[30] particularly among women with hypertensive disorders of pregnancy (HDP): there is a significant interaction between race/ethnicity and HDP for the outcome of maternal stroke during delivery hospitalization, with non-Hispanic blacks, Hispanics, and Asian/Pacific Islander women with HDP having more than double the risk of stroke compared with their white counterparts.[6] This difference is even larger when hemorrhagic stroke (ICH and SAH) is considered separately: black and Hispanic mothers with chronic hypertension had more than 6 times the risk of hemorrhagic stroke compared with white mothers with chronic hypertension.[6] A follow-up study found that the risk of ICH remained elevated up to 12 weeks postpartum with risk more than doubled in non-white groups.[31]

Although administrative data may provide important population-level insights related to disparities, major knowledge gaps remain. It is only partially understood to what degree patient factors, hospital factors, and provider factors account for adverse outcomes. There are limited population-level analyses incorporating longitudinal patient factors, which may more robustly adjust for case mix than cross-sectional data. Hospital factors in particular may play an important role in maternal disparities. Delivery in hospitals that serve high proportions of black obstetric patients are associated with higher risk of severe morbidity, even after risk adjustment.[16] In evaluating indicators of obstetric quality, research has found that black-serving hospitals perform poorly compared with white-serving and/or Hispanic-serving hospitals.[16,32] However, for many disparities analyses, evaluating hospital factors granularity is limited and data on resources and facilities, safety protocols, staffing, and other key attributes are not included. It is possible that the population of black-serving hospitals could overlap with the population of urban safety net hospitals providing care to a high acuity population and that with further risk adjustment and case-mix adjustment the effect of black-serving hospitals could be attenuated.

CLINICAL INFERENCES FROM MATERNAL DISPARITIES ADMINISTRATIVE DATA RESEARCH

A key clinical inference from the findings in administrative data research described earlier is that failure to rescue may represent an important contributor to maternal disparities. Failure to rescue is defined as a failure to prevent a clinically important deterioration, such as death or permanent disability, from a complication or an underlying illness or a complication of medical care.[33–37] The fact that non-Hispanic black women are at only modestly increased risk for common conditions such as preeclampsia and postpartum hemorrhage and that they are at much higher risk for death and major events leading to lifelong disability when these conditions are present supports the importance of failure to rescue in disparities, as does increased risk for preventable complications such as stroke.[3–6] Maternal mortality reviews support that deaths from hemorrhage and hypertension, increased among non-Hispanic black women in administrative data, are often preventable.[38] These findings underscore the importance of optimization of hospital-level strategies to reduce maternal risk such as implementation of safety bundles and interventions, which have been shown to be associated with decreased maternal risk for morbidity and mortality.[39–42] Although safety bundles may not explicitly address maternal risk by race, they do provide clear strategies to reduce risk from failure to rescue by, for example, administering antihypertensives in a timely manner and promptly recognizing and responding to obstetric hemorrhage. Given that non-Hispanic black women experience disproportionate risk in these clinical scenarios it is highly likely that they will benefit to a greater degree from risk reduction with care improvements.

A second key clinical inference from administrative data research is that given that risk is differential across conditions, it is highly likely that underlying health conditions play a major role in disparities. For example, black non-Hispanic women are at particularly high risk for cardiovascular complications, and it is unclear if there is any obstetric intervention that can reduce cardiovascular events. It is unlikely that for outcomes such as cardiovascular events addressing hospital level factors alone will be adequate in obviating differentials. Because cardiovascular and noncardiovascular medical conditions account for an even larger proportion of maternal mortality,[1] formalizing clinical recommendations for subspecialty care before, during, and after pregnancy for women with chronic conditions and new diagnoses made during pregnancy will represent an increasingly important component of strategies to decrease disparities. Obstetricians and obstetric clinical leadership may have opportunities to identify medical and other nonobstetrical subspecialists and to arrange follow-up to ensure that at-risk patients have optimal longitudinal care.

SUMMARY

Maternal disparities in the United States are increasingly well characterized, with non-Hispanic black women accounting for the largest attributable risk differential of any racial or ethnic group. A broad range of explanations and causality for maternal disparities have been proposed with conceptual frameworks imported from fields as diverse as sociology and social psychology.[43,44] Clinicians and clinical leaders are tasked with prioritizing interventions that (1) are feasible and implementable and (2) have a high likelihood, based on empirical evidence, of reducing risk. Although many knowledge gaps related to maternal disparities remain, findings from administrative data provide supporting evidence for 2 broad clinical inferences related to maternal disparities. First, failure to rescue in terms of both death and severe maternal morbidity (such as stroke in the setting of preeclampsia) likely account for a significant proportion of maternal disparities. Improving safety for leading conditions of maternal mortality such as preeclampsia and postpartum hemorrhage with safety bundles benefits all women but may benefit non-Hispanic black women most of all. Second, risk for adverse outcomes by race is generally differential with risk for some conditions similar for non-Hispanic black compared with other women but with large differences for others. These differentials including disproportionate cardiovascular risk support that underlying health conditions may represent an important contributor to overall disparities. Although future research is needed to disaggregate the contributions to racial disparities of patient, provider, and hospital factors and to determine how specific race-specific differentials can be mitigated, clinicians and clinical leaderships have major opportunities to improve care by reducing failure to rescue and improving longitudinal subspecialty care.

DISCLOSURES

Dr. Friedman is supported by the Health Resources and Services Administration Maternal and Child Health Bureau (R40 MC3287901).

REFERENCES

1. Creanga AA, Syverson C, Seed K, et al. Pregnancy-related mortality in the United States, 2011-2013. Obstet Gynecol 2017;130(2):366–73.
2. Petersen EE, Davis NL, Goodman D, et al. Racial/ethnic disparities in pregnancy-related deaths - United States, 2007-2016. MMWR Morb Mortal Wkly Rep 2019; 68(35):762–5.
3. Aziz A, Gyamfi-Bannerman C, Siddiq Z, et al. Maternal outcomes by race during postpartum readmissions. Am J Obstet Gynecol 2019;220(5):484.e1–10.
4. Gyamfi-Bannerman C, Pandita A, Miller EC, et al. Preeclampsia outcomes at delivery and race. J Matern Fetal Neonatal Med 2020;33(21):3619–26.
5. Gyamfi-Bannerman C, Srinivas SK, Wright JD, et al. Postpartum hemorrhage outcomes and race. Am J Obstet Gynecol 2018;219(2):185.e1–10.
6. Miller EC, Zambrano Espinoza MD, Huang Y, et al. Maternal race/ethnicity, hypertension, and risk for stroke during delivery admission. J Am Heart Assoc 2020; 9(3):e014775.
7. Grimes DA. Epidemiologic research using administrative databases: garbage in, garbage out. Obstet Gynecol 2010;116(5):1018–9.
8. Grimes DA. Epidemiologic research with administrative databases: red herrings, false alarms and pseudo-epidemics. Hum Reprod 2015;30(8):1749–52.
9. Healthcare cost and utilization Project. Overview of the national (nationwide) inpatient sample (NIS). Available at: https://www.hcup-us.ahrq.gov/nisoverview. jsp. Accessed July 10, 2020.
10. Healthcare cost and utilization Project. HCUP-US databases. Available at: https:// www.hcup-us.ahrq.gov/databases.jsp. Accessed July 10, 2020.
11. Bateman BT, Huybrechts KF, Hernandez-Diaz S, et al. Methylergonovine maleate and the risk of myocardial ischemia and infarction. Am J Obstet Gynecol 2013; 209(5):459.e1–3.
12. Cozowicz C, Olson A, Poeran J, et al. Opioid prescription levels and postoperative outcomes in orthopedic surgery. Pain 2017;158(12):2422–30.
13. Zilberberg MD, Nathanson BH, Sulham K, et al. Carbapenem resistance, inappropriate empiric treatment and outcomes among patients hospitalized with Enterobacteriaceae urinary tract infection, pneumonia and sepsis. BMC Infect Dis 2017;17(1):279.
14. Mardy AH, Siddiq Z, Ananth CV, et al. Venous thromboembolism prophylaxis during antepartum admissions and postpartum readmissions. Obstet Gynecol 2017; 130(2):270–8.
15. The Truven health MarketScan databases for Life Sciences researchers. Available at: https://truvenhealth.com/Portals/0/Assets/2017-MarketScan-Databases-Life-Sciences-Researchers-WP.pdf. Accessed January 21, 2019.
16. Howell EA, Egorova N, Balbierz A, et al. Black-white differences in severe maternal morbidity and site of care. Am J Obstet Gynecol 2015;214(1):122.e1–7.
17. Clowse ME, Grotegut C. Racial and ethnic disparities in the pregnancies of women with systemic lupus erythematosus. Arthritis Care Res (Hoboken) 2016; 68(10):1567–72.

18. Klemmensen AK, Olsen SF, Osterdal ML, et al. Validity of preeclampsia-related diagnoses recorded in a national hospital registry and in a postpartum interview of the women. Am J Epidemiol 2007;166(2):117–24.

19. Fang MC, Fan D, Sung SH, et al. Validity of using inpatient and outpatient administrative codes to identify acute venous thromboembolism: the CVRN VTE Study. Med Care 2017;55(12):e137–43.

20. James AH, Jamison MG, Brancazio LR, et al. Venous thromboembolism during pregnancy and the postpartum period: incidence, risk factors, and mortality. Am J Obstet Gynecol 2006;194(5):1311–5.

21. White RH, Brickner LA, Scannell KA. ICD-9-CM codes poorly identified venous thromboembolism during pregnancy. J Clin Epidemiol 2004;57(9):985–8.

22. White RH, Garcia M, Sadeghi B, et al. Evaluation of the predictive value of ICD-9-CM coded administrative data for venous thromboembolism in the United States. Thromb Res 2010;126(1):61–7.

23. Martin JN Jr, Thigpen BD, Moore RC, et al. Stroke and severe preeclampsia and eclampsia: a paradigm shift focusing on systolic blood pressure. Obstet Gynecol 2005;105(2):246–54.

24. Katsuragi S, Tanaka H, Hasegawa J, et al. Analysis of preventability of stroke-related maternal death from the nationwide registration system of maternal deaths in Japan. J Matern Fetal Neonatal Med 2018;31(16):2097–104.

25. Swartz RH, Cayley ML, Foley N, et al. The incidence of pregnancy-related stroke: a systematic review and meta-analysis. Int J Stroke 2017;12(7):687–97.

26. Miller EC, Gatollari HJ, Too G, et al. Risk factors for pregnancy-associated stroke in women with preeclampsia. Stroke 2017;48(7):1752–9.

27. Bateman BT, Schumacher HC, Bushnell CD, et al. Intracerebral hemorrhage in pregnancy: frequency, risk factors, and outcome. Neurology 2006;67(3):424–9.

28. Liang ZW, Lin L, Gao WL, et al. A clinical characteristic analysis of pregnancy-associated intracranial haemorrhage in China. Sci Rep 2015;5:9509.

29. Foo L, Bewley S, Rudd A. Maternal death from stroke: a thirty year national retrospective review. Eur J Obstet Gynecol Reprod Biol 2013;171(2):266–70.

30. Leffert LR, Clancy CR, Bateman BT, et al. Patient characteristics and outcomes after hemorrhagic stroke in pregnancy. Circ Cardiovasc Qual Outcomes 2015; 8(6 Suppl 3):S170–8.

31. Meeks JR, Bambhrollya AB, Alex KM, et al. Association of primary intracerebral hemorrhage with pregnancy and the postpartum period. JAMA Netw Open 2020;3(4):e202769.

32. Creanga AA, Bateman BT, Mhyre JM, et al. Performance of racial and ethnic minority-serving hospitals on delivery-related indicators. Am J Obstet Gynecol 2014;211(6):647.e1–6.

33. Ghaferi AA, Osborne NH, Birkmeyer JD, et al. Hospital characteristics associated with failure to rescue from complications after pancreatectomy. J Am Coll Surg 2010;211(3):325–30.

34. Ghaferi AA, Birkmeyer JD, Dimick JB. Hospital volume and failure to rescue with high-risk surgery. Med Care 2011;49(12):1076–81.

35. Ghaferi AA, Birkmeyer JD, Dimick JB. Variation in hospital mortality associated with inpatient surgery. N Engl J Med 2009;361(14):1368–75.

36. Ghaferi AA, Birkmeyer JD, Dimick JB. Complications, failure to rescue, and mortality with major inpatient surgery in medicare patients. Ann Surg 2009;250(6): 1029–34.

37. Patient Safety Net, the Agency for Healthcare Research and Quality. Failure to rescue. Available at: https://psnet.ahrq.gov/primer/failure-rescue. Accessed May 10, 2020.
38. Callaghan WM. State-based maternal death reviews: assessing opportunities to alter outcomes. Am J Obstet Gynecol 2014;211(6):581–2.
39. Main EK, Goffman D, Scavone BM, et al. National partnership for maternal safety: consensus bundle on obstetric hemorrhage. Obstet Gynecol 2015;126(1): 155–62.
40. Bernstein PS, Martin JN Jr, Barton JR, et al. National partnership for maternal safety: consensus bundle on severe hypertension during pregnancy and the postpartum period. Obstet Gynecol 2017;130(2):347–57.
41. Cleary KL, Siddiq Z, Ananth CV, et al. Use of antihypertensive medications during delivery hospitalizations complicated by preeclampsia. Obstet Gynecol 2018; 131(3):441–50.
42. Lu MC. Reducing maternal mortality in the United States. JAMA 2018;320(12): 1237–8.
43. Greenwald AG, Kriger LH. Implicit bias: Scientific foundations. Calif Law Rev 2006;94(No. 4):945–67.
44. Alvidrez J, Castille D, Laude-Sharp M, et al. The national institute on minority health and health disparities research framework. Am J Public Health 2019; 109(S1):S16–20.

Opioid Use and Misuse in Pregnancy

Ben Shatil, DO, MPH[a], Ruth Landau, MD[b],*

KEYWORDS

- Opioid use disorder • Opioid use in pregnancy • Opioid overprescription
- Opioid-sparing multimodal analgesia • Postpartum analgesia

KEY POINTS

- The rate of pregnant women with an opioid use disorder has paralleled the general population, increasing by 127% from 1998 to 2011.
- Chronic in utero opioid exposure is associated with neonatal opioid withdrawal syndrome, gastroschisis, preterm births, and small for gestational age. Postpartum maternal opioid consumption can also reach the newborn via breastmilk, causing colic, constipation, and sedation.
- Pain must be treated effectively, and this should be a priority in pregnancy. In fact, untreated pain is associated with a risk of greater opioid use, postpartum depression, and development of persistent postpartum pain.
- Stepwise multimodal analgesia is an effective method of treating either acute or chronic pain while minimizing opioid consumption. Multimodal opioid-sparing analgesia combines medications with differing mechanisms of action, such as acetaminophen, alpha-$_2$ agonists (eg, clonidine, dexmedetomidine), and local anesthetics (intravenous lidocaine, or lidocaine patch), to potentiate analgesic effects of opioids while minimizing their side effects.
- A patient's history and genetics can alter their opioid metabolism, pain management, and risk of developing an opioid use disorder. Tailoring a pain regimen for a patient's anticipated needs, while explaining benefits and risks, allows a personalized approach to medical management, minimizing unwanted effects.

INTRODUCTION

Opioids can be beneficial for pain management during pregnancy and postpartum when used appropriately. However, opioids are often misused and incorrectly prescribed. The opioid epidemic in the United States and worldwide has now been well established, with the lay press widely covering opioid overdose deaths that are still

[a] Department of Anesthesiology, Emory University Hospital Midtown, 550 Peachtree Street Northeast, Atlanta, GA 30308, USA; [b] Department of Anesthesiology, Columbia University Irving Medical Center, CHONY North CHN-1123, 3959 Broadway, New York, NY 10032, USA
* Corresponding author.
E-mail address: rl262@cumc.columbia.edu

Clin Perinatol 47 (2020) 769–777
https://doi.org/10.1016/j.clp.2020.08.004
0095-5108/20/© 2020 Elsevier Inc. All rights reserved.
perinatology.theclinics.com

occurring at growing rates. On average, 130 Americans die every day from an opioid overdose.[1]

In the obstetric population, additional concerns besides the effects of acute or chronic opioid use are to be accounted for. Pregnancies associated with opioid use, abuse, or dependence have significantly higher rates of complications, such as neonatal opioid withdrawal syndrome (NOWS), intrauterine growth restriction, neural tube defects, stillbirth, increased maternal mortality, greater postpartum pain, and longer inpatient stays.[2] Intrapartum opioid use impacts maternal, fetal, and obstetric outcomes. Furthermore, postpartum use of opioids increases the maternal risk of abuse and addiction, and opioids cross into breastmilk, leading to neonatal respiratory depression and gastrointestinal complications. Despite this, the prevalence of pregnant patients with an opioid use disorder (OUD) has paralleled the general population, with a 127% increase from 1998 to 2011.[3] From 2014 to 2015, the rate of overdose deaths among pregnant women increased 20%, and 4 times as many infants were born with NOWS.[1] The solution to the opioid crisis begins with understanding the physiology of pain and educating both health care providers and patients. Implementation of stepwise opioid-sparing multimodal analgesia, tailoring of and judicious use of opioid prescriptions, and shared decision making are some solutions to the opioid crisis that are discussed here.

OPIOID USE IN THE PREGNANT POPULATION

Women who use opioids during pregnancy are often stigmatized and shamed, lending to subpar medical care and even higher rates of morbidity and mortality. In the 1980s, the outcry against "crack babies," referring to neonatal abstinence syndrome, led to further studies demonstrating that opioid addiction was not a state of poor morality, but rather a physiologic disease now defined by the *Diagnostic and Statistical Manual of Mental Disorders* (Fifth Edition).[4] Although many opioid-using pregnant patients misuse opioids or have an OUD, some are prescribed opioids for legitimate concerns. For example, sickle cell patients often have a high opioid requirement because of years of treating vasoocclusive crises with ischemic pain. Pregnancy offers a unique opportunity to have multiple encounters with women who might otherwise not seek regular medical care over a short period. It is critical to recognize the difference between medically necessary opioid use and opioid misuse during these visits and create an appropriate peripartum plan. An antenatal consultation with the obstetric anesthesiologist team is warranted to assist with peripartum planning for women using opioids, particularly long acting (eg, methadone), or those with agonist/antagonist properties (eg, buprenorphine) during pregnancy, or those with chronic pain disorders. Substance use disorders affect women across all racial and ethnic groups and all socioeconomic groups and affect women in rural, urban, and suburban populations. Therefore, the American College of Obstetrics and Gynecology recommends universal screening for substance use for all patients at the first perinatal visit.[5]

OPIOID EFFECTS ON THE FETUS AND NEONATE

Pregnant women present a unique scenario whereby the effects of opioid consumption can directly affect both themselves and the fetus or neonate. Chronic in utero opioid exposure is associated with NOWS, gastroschisis, preterm births, and small for gestational age. In 2014, the incidence of NOWS ranged from 0.7 cases per 1000 hospital births to 33.4 cases per 1000 hospital births, increasing 300% in 10 years and occurring nationally at a rate of 1 infant born with NOWS every 15 minutes.[6] Furthermore, children younger than 6 years old have a significantly higher risk (odds ratio [OR] 2.13) of developing conduct disorder, and children older than 6 years old have a significantly higher risk (OR 2.55) of developing attention-deficit/hyperactivity disorder.[2]

Postpartum maternal opioid consumption can also reach the newborn via breast-milk, causing colic, constipation, and sedation. Codeine, a weak analgesic and a pro-drug, should be avoided because mothers who are ultrarapid metabolizers (CYP2D6) will convert codeine to morphine at a faster rate, causing higher rates of neonatal sedation, apnea, and bradycardia.[7] Therefore, opioid-sparing multimodal analgesia is preferable for breastfeeding mothers. Neuraxial opioids, acetaminophen, and nonsteroidal anti-inflammatory medications levels are insignificant in breastmilk transfer.[8]

PAIN MANAGEMENT DURING PREGNANCY

Pain must be treated effectively and should be a priority in pregnancy (**Box 1**). In fact, untreated pain is associated with a risk of greater opioid use, postpartum depression, and development of persistent postpartum pain.[9] During pregnancy, acetaminophen, rather than opioids, should be used as first-line treatment for acute pain.[10] When opi-oids are prescribed to manage acute pain in pregnancy, the lowest effective dose to achieve satisfactory relief should be used. When opioids are required, however, a sin-gle opioid given for the shortest duration is preferred.

Patients with chronic pain or a history of opioid use may benefit from a multidisci-plinary antenatal consultation, which in addition to the obstetric, neonatology, and anesthesia care teams, may include the acute and or chronic pain team as well as addictionology team as deemed appropriate. If the patient takes less than 60 mg oral morphine (or equivalent) daily, weaning from opioids early in pregnancy may be feasible with appropriate counseling and follow-up. However, at larger doses,

---

Box 1
Best practices

What is the current practice?

Opioid use in pregnancy
    Best practice/guidelines/care path objectives:
- Stepwise opioid-sparing multimodal analgesia is the best way to manage pain.
- Prescribe opioids judiciously because the more opioids are prescribed, the more patients consume.
- Breastfeeding is recommended for opioid-using mothers.
- Individualize pain management protocols based on data and a discussion with the patient about expectations and needs.
- Share pain management decision making with the patient.

What changes in current practice are likely to improve outcome?

- Universal screening for patients at risk of an opioid use disorder.
- Avoid opioids for patients with an uncomplicated vaginal delivery.
- Use opioid-sparing multimodal analgesia for women who undergo cesarean deliveries or complicated vaginal deliveries.
- Refer patients with an opioid use disorder to the anesthesia team early in pregnancy for a peripartum consult.
- Educate all providers, including obstetricians, nurses, and physician assistants, about optimal opioid use and multimodal analgesia.

withdrawal symptoms are more likely, which threaten preterm labor.[10] The standard of care for patients with an OUD is enrollment into a medication-assisted treatment plan, which combines opioid substitution with either methadone (opioid agonist) or buprenorphine (partial opioid agonist) with behavioral therapy.[7]

POSTPARTUM PAIN MANAGEMENT

Stepwise multimodal analgesia is an effective method of treating either acute or chronic pain while minimizing opioid consumption. Multimodal opioid-sparing analgesia combines medications with differing mechanisms of action, such as acetaminophen, alpha-$_2$ agonists (eg, clonidine, dexmedetomidine), and local anesthetics (intravenous lidocaine, or lidocaine patch), to potentiate analgesic effects of opioids while minimizing their side effects.

Women who undergo cesarean deliveries or complicated vaginal deliveries are expected to have increased postpartum pain compared with women with straightforward vaginal deliveries, and a stepwise multimodal opioid-sparing approach is the best method of effectively treating postpartum pain.[8] Neuraxial morphine (spinal or epidural) and scheduled oral acetaminophen and nonsteroidal anti-inflammatory (ie, ibuprofen) medications are recommended for effective pain management for all women undergoing cesarean deliveries with neuraxial anesthesia.[8] Oral opioids (ie, oxycodone) may be given as needed for breakthrough pain; however, current recommendations suggest maximal daily doses not exceeding 30 mg oral oxycodone.[9] In addition, regional blocks (transversus abdominus plane, quadratus lumborum), oral gabapentin, or intravenous ketamine should be considered for women with a risk of severe postpartum pain or a higher opioid tolerance.[8]

For patients with an OUD, baseline systemic opioid doses should be continued to avoid peripartum maternal withdrawal, with additional multimodal pain medications for postpartum pain management. Maintaining neuraxial epidural analgesia for 48 to 72 hours is advocated, which may include epidural analgesia with local anesthetics (usually low concentration of bupivacaine) via continuous infusion or programmed epidural intermittent bolus followed by one or several doses of preservative-free epidural morphine.[11] The unrefuted benefits of preservative-free morphine (Duramorph) given either epidurally (typically a dose of 3 mg) or intrathecally (150–300 μg) are the prolonged analgesic effect (up to 24 hours after a single dose), and the improved analgesia compared with systemic opioids. Neuraxial morphine carries a lower risk for respiratory depression and other opioid-related side effects when compared with systemic opioids.[12] The Society for Obstetric Anesthesia and Perinatology promotes that with a single low dose of neuraxial morphine, it is appropriate to reduce the frequency and duration of respiratory monitoring in healthy mothers while focusing vigilance on monitoring in those women at highest risk for respiratory depression, such as those with sleep apnea or morbid obesity.[13] In addition, neuraxial opioids do not cross into the breastmilk, which reduces the risk of neonatal sedation and respiratory depression.

OPIOID MISUSE

Opioid misuse in pregnancy can have a ripple effect, causing multiple concerns with pain management, overdose, and addiction. Opioid users have a risk of developing *hyperalgesia* (**Table 1**), often causing incomplete peripartum analgesia and making postpartum pain management challenging.[14] The continuous opioid receptor site occupation by medications causes proliferation of opioid receptors such that minimal painful stimuli result in a hyperalgesic state, making acute pain significantly more

Table 1
Glossary of terms and conditions related to pain

Term	Definition
Pain	An unpleasant sensory and emotional experience associated with actual or potential tissue damage, or described in terms of such damage[29] A new definition has been proposed: An aversive sensory and emotional experience typically caused by, or resembling that caused by, actual or potential tissue injury[30]
Acute pain	Pain that is usually sharp and severe, may start suddenly, and has a known cause, like an injury or surgery, and typically lasts <3 mo[31]
Allodynia	Pain due to a stimulus that does not typically provoke pain[32]
Analgesia	Absence of pain in response to stimulation that would normally be painful
Chronic pain	Pain that lasts 3 mo or more and can be caused by a disease or condition, injury, medical treatment, inflammation, or an unknown reason[31]
Dysesthesia	An unpleasant abnormal sensation, whether spontaneous or evoked
Hyperalgesia	Increased painful response either to a less painful stimulus or at a lower pain threshold. Current evidence suggests that hyperalgesia is a consequence of perturbation of the nociceptive system with peripheral or central sensitization, or both[32]
Hyperpathia	A painful syndrome characterized by an abnormally painful reaction to a stimulus, especially a repetitive stimulus, as well as an increased threshold
Opioid dependence	The body's adaptation to an opioid that produces symptoms of withdrawal when the drug is stopped[31]
Opioid-induced hyperalgesia	A state of nociceptive sensitization caused by exposure to opioids characterized by a paradoxic response whereby a patient receiving opioids for the treatment of pain could actually become more sensitive to certain painful stimuli and experience atypical pain[33]
Opioid tolerance	A need for increased amount of opioids or a diminished effect with the same amount[34]
Opioid use disorder	Defined as having at least two of the following within a 12-mo period: (1) taking larger amounts of opioids than intended or for longer than intended, (2) either persistent desire or unsuccessful attempts to stop opioid use, (3) spending a significant amount of time looking for opioids or recovering from their effects, (4) craving opioids, (5) problems fulfilling obligations, (6) continued opioid use despite interpersonal problems, (7) giving up activities due to opioid use, (8) using opioids in physically hazardous situations, (9) continued opioid use despite physical or psychological problem, (10) tolerance, or (11) experiencing withdrawal symptoms or taking opioids to avoid withdrawal symptoms[34]

difficult to manage.[15] Thus, a *tolerance* to the analgesic effects of opioids develops, and higher doses are required to achieve adequate analgesia. However, opioid tolerance does not protect from the sedative effects of opioids. These patients are almost equally as susceptible to oversedation and respiratory depression as a non-opioid-using pregnant woman, increasing risk of overdose-related death.[3] Morbid obesity, obstructive sleep apnea, and concomitant use of benzodiazepines also exacerbate opioid-induced respiratory depression. Patients on methadone, an NMDA receptor antagonist and alpha-adrenergic agonist, may not develop pronounced opioid tolerance or hyperalgesia.[15,16]

Opioids are often misused and abused, leading to *dependence* and addiction. A recent study reported that 1 in 300 opioid-naïve women will become dependent on opioids after a cesarean delivery.[17] Patients with a history of substance abuse, patients who smoke tobacco, or those taking antidepressant medications are at a higher risk of becoming persistent users. A multimodal opioid-sparing approach minimizes this risk significantly by reducing inpatient consumption and the need for opioids on discharge. Obstetricians should carefully consider alternatives before prescribing opioids at discharge because of the risk of dependence and the effect these drugs can have on parenting safety.[10] Physical dependence can develop as quickly as 4 to 8 weeks, varying based on the patient's history of opioid use, and other genetic and environmental factors.[18]

EFFECTS OF OVERPRESCRIPTION OF OPIOIDS

With the knowledge of the opioid epidemic, health care providers should ensure that opioids are always appropriately indicated, consider nonopioid alternatives, and prescribe opioids judiciously. The Center for Disease Control and Prevention published an "opioid-prescribing guideline" that promotes setting realistic pain management goals with patients, using nonopioid alternatives, and close follow-up.[19] The more opioids given during postpartum hospital stay directly correlates to a greater opioid use after discharge. Likewise, the more opioids prescribed at discharge, the more opioids that are consumed postpartum. Despite higher opioid consumption, pain scores and patient satisfaction rates did not differ from patients taking no opioids.[20]

Currently, postpartum opioids are exceedingly overprescribed. One study reported that 89% of women who undergo a cesarean delivery and 52.7% of women who had a vaginal delivery filled an opioid prescription at discharge.[21] Similarly, another study reported that 85.4% of women filled an opioid prescription after cesarean section, receiving an average of 40 pills. From that cohort, the median number of pills consumed was 20, leaving 20 pills unused, and 95.3% of women did not dispose of their leftover opioids.[22] Leftovers are at risk of diversion and abuse, worsening the opioid epidemic.

A TAILORED APPROACH TO SHARED DECISION MAKING FOR PAIN MANAGEMENT

A patient's history and genetics can alter their opioid metabolism, pain management, and risk of developing an OUD. Variants in the mu-opioid and dopamine genes are associated with differing responses to exogenous opioid consumption and the risk of developing an OUD.[23] Therefore, it is reasonable to claim that standardized pain order sets are not suited for every patient. Some women may be undertreated, and left in pain, whereas others may be overtreated and are at greater risk of experiencing unwanted side effects. Preoperative pain prediction tools, such as assessing pain score with local anesthetic infiltration and asking women about their anticipated pain and relief, may assist in planning postpartum pain management.[24] Tailoring a pain regimen for a patient's anticipated needs, while explaining benefits and risks, allows a personalized approach to medical management, minimizing unwanted effects.

Varying clinical scenarios also influence the amount of pain and need for more complex pain management. Patients with uncomplicated vaginal deliveries, for example, experience a median of 14 days to pain resolution, with pain scores in the mild to moderate range, and require no opioids for pain management.[25] However, opioids are often prescribed to patients after vaginal delivery. Unscheduled cesarean delivery (ie, intrapartum) is suggested to increase postoperative opioid use compared with a scheduled cesarean delivery.[26] Furthermore, women with a longer labor course before proceeding to an intrapartum cesarean delivery may likely have increased postpartum pain and a higher risk of requiring opioids for breakthrough pain.[27] A previous cesarean delivery with residual scar hyperalgesia is also thought to increase analgesic use, because of central hypersensitization.[28] Other important factors to consider are obstructive sleep apnea, contraindications to neuraxial, and a history of OUD. With the assistance of such data, the physician should set realistic expectations and allow the patient to share in decision making by discussing preferences for pain relief and for avoidance of side effects after cesarean delivery.[24] A tailored pain management protocol reached by shared patient-physician decision making can reduce unnecessary opioid analgesic consumption and might be part of the solution to the opioid epidemic.

SUMMARY

It is the responsibility of clinicians to practice the best, up-to-date evidence-based medicine and advocate for the patient. Although only 1 in 300 opioid-naïve women may become persistent opioid users and dependent, that equates to more than 21,000 new chronic opioid users annually after childbirth.[17,21] Patient education about the risks and benefits of multimodal analgesia and empowering shared decision making can help curb the epidemic. Tailoring pain management to individual needs might be a solution to the problem.

CLINICS CARE POINTS

- The obstetrician often has a unique advantage of screening the patient for a substance use disorder early in pregnancy and should do so in the first prenatal visit per ACOG guidelines.
- Patients with a known or suspected opioid use disorder should have a multidisciplinary antenatal consultation with obstetrics, neonatology, and anesthesiology care teams.
- Untreated pain is associated with a greater risk of opioid use, postpartum depression, and the development of pesistent postpartum pain. Appropriate pain management, using opioid-sparing multimodal analgesia, should always be utilized.

DISCLOSURE

There are no commercial or financial conflicts of interest to disclose. There were no required funding sources.

REFERENCES

1. CDC. Opioid overdose: understanding the epidemic. Centers for Disease Control and Prevention. 2018. Available at: https://www.cdc.gov/drugoverdose/epidemic/index.html. Accessed March 12, 2020.
2. Azuine RE, Ji Y, Chang HY, et al. Prenatal risk factors and perinatal and postnatal outcomes associated with maternal opioid exposure in an urban, low-income, multiethnic US population. JAMA Netw Open 2019;2(6):e196405.
3. Maeda A, Bateman BT, Clancy CR, et al. Opioid abuse and dependence during pregnancy: temporal trends and obstetrical outcomes. Anesthesiology 2014; 121(6):1158–65.

4. Tauger N. Opioid dependence and pregnancy in early twentieth-century America. Addiction 2018;113(5):952–7.
5. Committee opinion No. 711 summary: opioid use and opioid use disorder in pregnancy. Obstet Gynecol 2017;130(2):488–9.
6. CDC. Evaluation of state-mandated reporting of neonatal abstinence syndrome — six states, 2013–2017. Centers for Disease Control and Prevention. 2019. Available at: https://www.cdc.gov/mmwr/volumes/68/wr/mm6801a2.htm. Accessed May 13, 2020.
7. Ordean A, Wong S, Graves L. No. 349-Substance use in pregnancy. J Obstet Gynaecol Can 2017;39(10):922–937 e922.
8. Carvalho B, Butwick AJ. Postcesarean delivery analgesia. Best Pract Res Clin Anaesthesiol 2017;31(1):69–79.
9. ACOG committee opinion No. 742: postpartum pain management. Obstet Gynecol 2018;132(1):e35–43.
10. Blandthorn J, Leung L, Loke Y, et al. Prescription opioid use in pregnancy. Aust N Z J Obstet Gynaecol 2018;58(5):494–8.
11. Landau R. Post-cesarean delivery pain. Management of the opioid-dependent patient before, during and after cesarean delivery. Int J Obstet Anesth 2019; 39:105–16.
12. Yurashevich M, Habib AS. Monitoring, prevention and treatment of side effects of long-acting neuraxial opioids for post-cesarean analgesia. Int J Obstet Anesth 2019;39:117–28.
13. Bauchat JR, Weiniger CF, Sultan P, et al. Society for Obstetric Anesthesia and Perinatology consensus statement: monitoring recommendations for prevention and detection of respiratory depression associated with administration of neuraxial morphine for cesarean delivery analgesia. Anesth Analg 2019;129(2):458–74.
14. Cassidy B, Cyna AM. Challenges that opioid-dependent women present to the obstetric anaesthetist. Anaesth Intensive Care 2004;32(4):494–501.
15. Mitra S, Sinatra RS. Perioperative management of acute pain in the opioid-dependent patient. Anesthesiology 2004;101(1):212–27.
16. Higgins C, Smith BH, Matthews K. Evidence of opioid-induced hyperalgesia in clinical populations after chronic opioid exposure: a systematic review and meta-analysis. Br J Anaesth 2019;122(6):e114–26.
17. Bateman BT, Franklin JM, Bykov K, et al. Persistent opioid use following cesarean delivery: patterns and predictors among opioid-naive women. Am J Obstet Gynecol 2016;215(3):353.e1-18.
18. Association AP. Opioid use disorder. American Psychiatric Association. 2018. Available at: https://www.psychiatry.org/patients-families/addiction/opioid-use-disorder/opioid-use-disorder. Accessed May 13, 2020.
19. Frieden TR, Houry D. Reducing the risks of relief–the CDC opioid-prescribing guideline. N Engl J Med 2016;374(16):1501–4.
20. Komatsu R, Ando K, Flood PD. Factors associated with persistent pain after childbirth: a narrative review. Br J Anaesth 2020;124(3):e117–30.
21. Osmundson SS, Wiese AD, Min JY, et al. Delivery type, opioid prescribing, and the risk of persistent opioid use after delivery. Am J Obstet Gynecol 2019; 220(4):405–7.
22. Bateman BT, Cole NM, Maeda A, et al. Patterns of opioid prescription and use after cesarean delivery. Obstet Gynecol 2017;130(1):29–35.
23. Crist RC, Reiner BC, Berrettini WH. A review of opioid addiction genetics. Curr Opin Psychol 2019;27:31–5.

24. Carvalho B, Habib AS. Personalized analgesic management for cesarean delivery. Int J Obstet Anesth 2019;40:91–100.
25. Komatsu R, Carvalho B, Flood PD. Recovery after nulliparous birth: a detailed analysis of pain analgesia and recovery of function. Anesthesiology 2017; 127(4):684–94.
26. Prabhu M, Dolisca S, Wood R, et al. Postoperative opioid consumption after scheduled compared with unscheduled cesarean delivery. Obstet Gynecol 2019;133(2):354–63.
27. Shatil BS, Daoud B, Guglielminotti J, et al. Association between opioid use after intrapartum cesarean delivery and repeat cesarean delivery: a retrospective cohort study. Int J Obstet Anesth 2020;42:120–2.
28. Ortner CM, Granot M, Richebe P, et al. Preoperative scar hyperalgesia is associated with post-operative pain in women undergoing a repeat caesarean delivery. Eur J Pain 2013;17(1):111–23.
29. Treede RD. The International Association for the Study of Pain definition of pain: as valid in 2018 as in 1979, but in need of regularly updated footnotes. Pain Rep 2018;3(2):e643.
30. Available at: https://www.iasp-pain.org/PublicationsNews/NewsDetail.aspx?ItemNumber=9218. Accessed May 30, 2020.
31. CDC. Opioid overdose. Center for Disease Control and Prevention. 2020. Available at: https://www.cdc.gov/drugoverdose/opioids/terms.html. Accessed May 13, 2020.
32. IASP. IASP terminology. International Association for the Study of Pain. 2017. Available at: https://www.iasp-pain.org/Education/Content.aspx?ItemNumber=1698. Accessed May 13, 2020.
33. Lee M, Silverman SM, Hansen H, et al. A comprehensive review of opioid-induced hyperalgesia. Pain Physician 2011;14(2):145–61.
34. Association AP. Diagnostic and statistical manual of mental disorders (DSM–5). American Psychiatric Association. Available at: https://www.psychiatry.org/psychiatrists/practice/dsm. Accessed May 13, 2020.

Advances in Maternal Fetal Medicine

Perinatal Quality Collaboratives Working Together to Improve Maternal Outcomes

Patricia Ann Lee King, PhD, MSW[a,b], Zsakeba T. Henderson, MD[c],
Ann E.B. Borders, MD, MSc, MPH[a,b,d],*

KEYWORDS

- Perinatal quality collaboratives • Quality improvement • Maternal mortality
- Birth equity • Maternal outcomes

KEY POINTS

- Perinatal quality collaboratives (PQCs) are an effective intervention to improve maternal health outcomes.
- Physician, nursing, and public health champions provide leadership for effective quality improvement initiatives, optimally engage hospital teams, and achieve sustainable improvements in care.
- Given the urgent challenges facing maternal and newborn health across the country, an emphasis on developing and sustaining PQCs nationwide is needed.
- Promotion of partnerships at the federal, state, and local levels is important to ensure effective collaboration to address the urgent need to improve maternal health.

Disclaimer: The findings and conclusions in this article are those of the authors and do not necessarily represent the official position of the Centers for Disease Control and Prevention.
[a] Feinberg School of Medicine, Center for HealthCare Services and Outcomes Research, Institute for Public Health and Medicine, Northwestern University, 633 North St. Clair, 20th Floor, Chicago, IL 60611, USA; [b] Pritzker School of Medicine, University of Chicago, Chicago, IL, USA; [c] Division of Reproductive Health, NCCDPHP, Centers for Disease Control and Prevention, 4770 Buford Highway Northeast, MS S107-2, Atlanta, GA 30341-3724, USA; [d] Division of Maternal-Fetal Medicine, Department of Obstetrics and Gynecology, NorthShore University HealthSystem, 2650 Ridge Avenue, Evanston, IL 60201, USA
* Corresponding author. Division of Maternal-Fetal Medicine, Department of Obstetrics and Gynecology, NorthShore University HealthSystem, 2650 Ridge Avenue, Evanston, IL 60201.
E-mail address: info@ilpqc.org

Clin Perinatol 47 (2020) 779–797
https://doi.org/10.1016/j.clp.2020.08.009
0095-5108/20/© 2020 Elsevier Inc. All rights reserved.

perinatology.theclinics.com

INTRODUCTION

Despite many advances in evidence-based perinatal care, perinatal health outcomes in the United States are suboptimal.[1–4] While national maternal mortality rates are decreasing in many countries, they continue to rise in the U.S.[1] and infant mortality rates in the U.S. are greater than in many other developed countries.[2,3] There are also persistent racial-ethnic disparities in both infant and maternal outcomes.[2,4] There are ongoing efforts across the country to address these urgent challenges in perinatal health and improve outcomes. State-based perinatal quality collaboratives (PQCs) have shown that the application of collaborative improvement science methods can optimize perinatal health outcomes.[5] PQCs are state or multistate networks that improve measurable outcomes for maternal and infant health by advancing evidence-informed clinical practices and processes using quality improvement (QI) strategies. They address gaps by working with clinical teams, public health leaders, and other stakeholders, including patients and families, to implement statewide initiatives that spread best clinical practices, reduce variation in practice, and promote health equity.[5]

PQCs represent a community of change, identifying health care processes that need to be improved and using the best available methods to make changes as quickly as possible.[6] The PQC model of perinatal QI has shown success in rapid scale-up of evidence-based practices by leveraging state and local stakeholders.[6] They engage clinical hospital teams into a network that shares ideas, tools, and strategies for implementation of improvement projects and initiatives. There is growing evidence of how PQCs have contributed to important changes in perinatal health care and how their work has led to significant improvements in perinatal outcomes.

PQCs are now developing across the country and are making progress in improving maternal health outcomes, as will be described later. Sustaining this progress will take improved awareness of the important role of PQCs in this effort and the need for ongoing support and collaboration. This article describes PQC history, infrastructure and function, and the role of obstetric providers in PQC work, as well as providing examples of progress and successes PQCs have achieved to improve maternal care and outcomes.

THE HISTORY OF PERINATAL QUALITY COLLABORATIVES

The number of PQCs in the United States has grown considerably over the last decade, with almost every state currently having an active PQC or one in development.[5,7] However, the road to building statewide capacity to improve perinatal care has been a long one. In the 1990s, the Institute of Medicine (IOM) put new emphasis on QI that led to the publication of 2 reports that fixed national attention on the critical need for QI in health care.[8,9] In the 2001 report, "Crossing the Quality Chasm," the IOM charged the health care system with frequently lacking "the environment, the processes, and the capabilities needed to ensure that services are safe, effective, patient-centered, timely, efficient, and equitable,"[9] qualities called the "six aims for improvement."[9] In addition to achieving these aims, the IOM recommended improving patient safety and reducing medical error by establishing a national focus on leadership, research, tools, and protocols about safety.[9,10] Over the next decade, many organizations, including private and professional organizations, along with federal and state governments responded, and were instrumental in guiding the evolution of the perinatal system of care and early QI efforts. This included work by the Institute of Healthcare Improvement (IHI) that spearheaded the use of collaborative quality improvement; the first formal improvement collaborative in neonatology conducted by the Vermont Oxford Network; and regional collaborative improvement work in neonatology.[6,10] This work was followed by a focus on quality of care for mothers and newborns by multiple professional organizations that led to new quality measures and standards for improving maternity care.[10,11]

The increased growth of PQCs is largely caused by the work and support received from state and national programs to build capacity and infrastructure for PQCs. Since 2011, the Centers for Disease Control and Prevention (CDC) has supported state PQCs and currently provides funding for 13 state PQCs and the National Network of Perinatal Quality Collaboratives (NNPQC). The NNPQC was launched in 2016 in coordination with the March of Dimes and is now coordinated by the National Institute for Children's Health Quality (NICHQ). The NNPQC provides technical support for PQCs, identifying and disseminating best practices for establishing and sustaining all PQCs across the country.[5] Another important source of resources and support for PQCs has been the Alliance for Innovation on Maternal Health (AIM). In 2014, AIM was funded by the Health Resources and Services Administration (HRSA) to develop maternal safety bundles of evidence-based practices that are implemented statewide by PQCs.[5,12]

PERINATAL QUALITY COLLABORATIVE INFRASTRUCTURE AND FUNCTION

Although there are many state-based organizations that address issues of perinatal care, PQCs serve a specific role in using data and QI methods to make measurable improvements in care and outcomes. Many PQCs use the IHI Breakthrough Series model to implement QI science at the collaborative level (**Fig. 1**).[13] Key strategies used by PQCs include (1) collaborative learning to provide opportunities for clinical teams across the state to share knowledge, strategies, and experiences while working toward unified objectives for improvement; (2) use of rapid-response data with regular data reports for clinical teams to monitor progress across time and compare progress with other teams toward meeting those objectives; and (3) provision of QI science support and assistance to clinical teams (**Fig. 2**).[5] The ultimate goal of PQCs is to achieve sustainable improvements in population-level outcomes in maternal and infant health. Clinical teams are the heart of a PQC, and they drive the processes and change that happens at the local level.

There are various organizational structures and homes for PQCs, with some being stand-alone organizations and other PQCs based in organizations such as academic institutions, state health departments, state Medicaid programs, or state hospital associations.[5] Despite the variety in organizational structure, the following key roles are central to all PQCs[14]: (1) successful PQCs have both maternal and neonatal clinical leadership to provide input for initiatives and to champion efforts among clinical providers; (2) QI experts are critical for providing QI assistance and support to clinical teams and for helping to plan and execute improvement projects; (3) a data lead or data team who is responsible for overseeing data collection systems, data management, analysis, and data reports is also crucial; (4) a program/project manager or coordinator manages the daily PQC activities, such as securing engagement of clinical teams, stakeholders, and partners; managing resource development, collaborative learning webinars, and in-person meetings; and fiscal oversight. Although funding for staffing of a PQC has been reported as a major challenge by many PQCs,[5] it is crucial that key roles and responsibilities are clear and that there is a mechanism for stakeholders to provide regular input to the work. It is also important that initiatives are implemented across participating hospitals with key aims and strategies identified. Hospital teams must be engaged, supported, and provided with timely data reporting

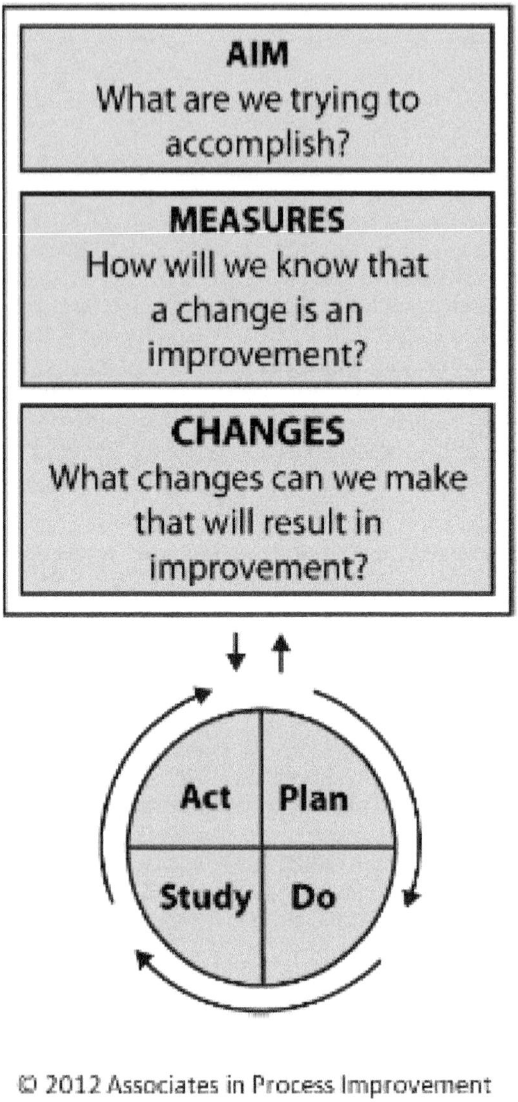

Fig. 1. The model for improvement. (*From* Langley GL MR, Nolan TW, Norman CL, Provost LP. The improvement guide: a practical approach to enhancing organizational performance 2nd ed. San Fransico: Jossey-Bass Publishers; 2009; with permission.)

on key measures to drive the QI work and ultimately achieve sustainable improvements in care and outcomes.[14]

The work of PQCs involves many partners and complements other programs for synergistic impact on maternal health (**Fig. 3**). PQCs have partnered with AIM to support implementation of AIM maternal safety bundles at the state level through statewide hospital QI initiatives. The AIM maternal safety bundles are an important source of resources and toolkit material for PQCs.[15] As state maternal mortality committees (MMRCs) have expanded across the country, PQCs are more frequently

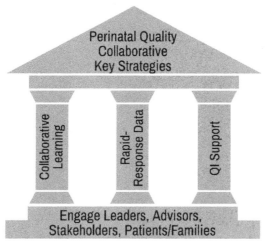

Fig. 2. Key strategies used by PQCs. (*Adapted from* Lee King PA, Young D, Borders AEB. A framework to harness the power of quality collaboratives to improve perinatal outcomes. Clinical Obstetrics and Gynecology. 2019;62(3):606; with permission.)

collaborating with MMRCs to use data and prevention recommendations to implement and scale up interventions for statewide, population-level improvements. This process includes using review data to prioritize and tailor initiatives on the leading causes of maternal death in the state, and the recommendations to inform interventions for improvement in maternal and perinatal outcomes.[16,17]

THE ROLE OF MATERNAL-FETAL MEDICINE/OBSTETRIC PROVIDERS IN PERINATAL QUALITY COLLABORATIVE SUCCESS

Obstetric providers, including maternal-fetal medicine physicians, play a critical role in the success of PQCs. At the national level, the Society for Maternal-Fetal Medicine (SMFM) and the American College of Obstetricians and Gynecologists (ACOG) have recognized the importance of supporting QI leadership, advocacy, and research to improve maternal and pregnancy outcomes. The American Board of Obstetrics and

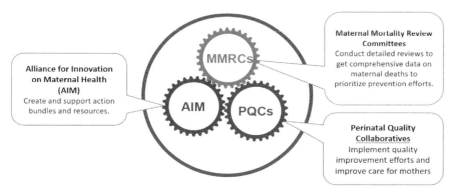

Fig. 3. The relationship between PQCs, maternal mortality committees (MMRCs), and AIM. *From* Goodman DA; Centers for Disease Control and Prevention. Safe motherhood: anupdate from CDC. Presented at the Title V Technical Assistance Meeting. Arlington, VA. October 15, 2018.

Gynecology (ABOG) has supported PQCs by awarding Maintenance of Certification credit for obstetric providers' participation in approved PQC QI initiatives. At the state level, PQCs are typically led by maternal-fetal medicine/obstetric champions in partnership with neonatal and nursing colleagues, as well as QI and public health leadership. Engagement of obstetric provider leaders at the state level is critical for PQC success. There are multiple roles for obstetric leaders at the PQC level, including (1) PQC leadership, (2) initiative leadership, (3) advisory workgroup membership, (4) grand rounds speakers bureau, and (5) participation in PQC in-person meetings (**Table 1**).[15]

Regardless of PQC leadership, improvement in maternal care and outcomes does not happen unless obstetric providers are engaged in QI leadership at the hospital level. Every clinical team working on an obstetric/maternal QI initiative must have an obstetric champion and a nursing champion to be successful. Challenges with engaging obstetric champions is one of the most common barriers reported by hospital teams that are struggling to achieve QI initiative aims.[14] Obstetric leaders at the state and hospital levels are instrumental for achieving provider buy-in and clinical culture change. At the clinical level, all obstetric providers can support QI initiative success by engaging in initiative education and actively supporting system and practice changes. It takes providers at all levels for PQCs to successfully improve maternal care and outcomes for all patients.

STATE PERINATAL QUALITY COLLABORATIVE IMPACT ON OBSTETRIC CARE AND OUTCOMES
Maternal Morbidity and Mortality

With maternal mortality rates not improving in the United States, maternal-fetal medicine leaders are calling for focused maternal improvement efforts to put the "M back into maternal-fetal medicine."[18] PQCs are acting on this call, resulting in most current initiatives focusing on identification and management of the primary causes of severe maternal morbidity (SMM) and mortality. Examples of successful maternal PQC initiatives addressing obstetric hemorrhage, severe maternal hypertension, maternal opioid use disorder (OUD), cardiovascular disease and venous thromboembolism, promotion of vaginal birth/safe reduction of primary cesarean section (CS), access to immediate postpartum long-acting reversible contraception (IPLARC), and access to postpartum care are discussed here.[19–57]

Table 1
Roles for obstetric leaders in perinatal quality collaboratives[15]

Roles for Obstetric Leaders	Description
PQC leadership	Provides overall clinical and/or executive leadership to the collaborative
Initiative leadership	Provides expert guidance for specific QI initiatives as an expert advisory panel member or clinical lead
Advisory workgroup member	Provides input on PQC and QI initiatives progress in regular meetings
Grand rounds speakers bureau	Shares QI initiative messages with hospitals across the state in as-needed presentations at hospitals
In-person meetings	Participates in collaborative in-person meetings, including breakout discussions

Data from Lee King PA, Young D, Borders AEB. A framework to harness the power of quality collaboratives to improve perinatal outcomes. Clinical Obstetrics and Gynecology. 2019;62(3):606.

Promoting vaginal birth initiatives

Cesarean delivery is associated with greater rates of maternal morbidity and mortality than vaginal delivery.[19] The cesarean delivery rate is a key quality indicator for obstetric care, and the US Office of Disease Prevention and Health Promotion's Healthy People 2020 goal of a nulliparous, transverse, singleton, vertex (NTSV) CS rate is 24.7% or less.[20,21] In 2014, ACOG published an obstetric care consensus on safe prevention of the primary cesarean delivery,[22] and, in 2015, AIM developed the Safe Reduction of Primary Cesarean Births bundle.[23]

The California Maternal Quality Care Collaborative (CMQCC) piloted a Supporting Vaginal Birth QI initiative with a toolkit and implementation guide in 2015 involving 3 hospitals, which resulted in an average 18.6% reduction in NTSV CS rates.[24,25] CMQCC then launched a statewide initiative and early cohorts included 56 hospitals with NTSV CS rates of more than 23.9%. Over the course of the collaborative, the NTSV CS rate decreased from 29.3% in 2015 to 25.0% in 2017 (adjusted odds ratio, 0.76; 95% confidence interval, 0.73–0.78) among participating hospitals with no adverse impact on maternal or neonatal safety.[26]

The Florida Perinatal Quality Collaborative (FPQC) Promoting Primary Vaginal Deliveries (PROVIDE) initiative launched in October 2017 and reduced the NTSV CS rate by 7% across 42 participating hospitals by 2019.[27] FPQC enhanced and expanded their initiative and launched PROVIDE 2.0 to 76 hospitals to continue work toward their aim of a 20% reduction across participating hospitals.[28,29] PQC initiatives to promote vaginal birth will support hospitals in achieving Healthy People 2020 goals.[21]

Postpartum hemorrhage

Postpartum hemorrhage is a leading cause of maternal mortality in the week after delivery and many of these deaths are preventable.[30,31] ACOG expanded guidance on postpartum hemorrhage to include recommendations for hospital-wide standard protocols and treatment algorithms.[32] AIM developed the Obstetric Hemorrhage bundle,[33] including resources from the ACOG District II Safe Motherhood Initiative bundle[34] and PQC-developed toolkits.[35,36] The FPQC Obstetric Hemorrhage Initiative ran from December 2013 to April 2015 and included 35 hospitals.[37] Participating hospitals improved, from baseline to the initiative end, across all process measures, including increasing clinical staff (100% trained) and provider education (71% trained), completion of risk assessment for obstetric hemorrhage (from 11% to 75%), documentation of active management of the third stage of labor (from 55% to 87%), and quantification of blood loss for vaginal deliveries (from 43% to 76%).[37] The FPQC found that obstetric and nursing leadership and staff buy-in, the strength of the evidence for treatment guidelines, adaptability of QI tools across hospital settings, and organization of the resources and collaborative support components contributed to successful hospital implementation.[38]

The CMQCC Obstetric Hemorrhage Initiative was conducted from January 2015 to March 2016 and reduced SMM among women with hemorrhage in 99 collaborative hospitals by 20.8% from baseline to the last half of the initiative.[39] The CMQCC showed that participating in a statewide collaborative postpartum hemorrhage QI initiative achieved a significantly greater reduction in SMM than was achieved in women with hemorrhage at hospitals not participating in the collaborative.[39]

Hypertensive disorders of pregnancy and the postpartum

Hypertensive disorders of pregnancy are another major cause of maternal mortality and many deaths are preventable.[30,31] ACOG provides current guidance on emergent therapy for acute-onset severe hypertension during pregnancy and the postpartum, which recommends urgent treatment (within 30–60 minutes) with anti-hypertensive therapy.[40] These recommendations are supported in the AIM Severe Hypertension in Pregnancy bundle.[41] The CMQCC's initial preeclampsia initiative launched in 2013 and lasted 2 years. There were 24 participating hospitals that achieved a 42% increase in treatment of severe hypertension, a 34% decrease in SMM overall, and 48% decrease in SMM excluding hemorrhage from baseline (6 months preinitiative) to the 6-month period 9 to 15 months after the start of the initiative.[42] CMQCC expanded this work through the California Partnership for Maternal Safety collaborative with 126 hospitals working from 2013 to 2016 to help implement CMQCC toolkits for a standard approach to preeclampsia and obstetric hemorrhage.[43]

The Illinois Perinatal Quality Collaborative (ILPQC) Severe Maternal Hypertension Initiative launched in May 2016 and lasted through December 2017 with 102 hospitals. Preliminary results in the first year of the initiative show an increased percentage of patients with new-onset severe hypertension treated within 60 minutes from 41% at baseline to 79% in the first year of the initiative,[44] with final results pending publication (Borders and colleagues, submitted for publication). Preliminary results also showed an increase in the percentage of cases receiving preeclampsia education at discharge, from 37% to 81%; scheduling follow-up appointments within 10 days of discharge, from 53% to 75%; and debrief after event, from 2% to 44%.[44] PQC initiatives to address severe maternal hypertension will support hospital work toward The Joint Commission Standards effective July 2020.[11,45]

Opioid use disorder in pregnancy

Maternal OUD at delivery more than quadrupled from 1999 to 2014.[46] Mental health and substance abuse are a leading cause of maternal death.[47] PQCs are working to help hospitals address variation in the quality of care for women with OUD in obstetric settings and during the delivery admission, including promotion of QI strategies that support implementation of national ACOG guidelines to improve maternal outcomes for women with OUD.[48] The AIM Obstetric Care for Women with OUD Bundle includes resources on screening, brief intervention with assessment of readiness for medication-assisted treatment (MAT) and referral to recovery treatment, obstetric care guidelines including pain management, naloxone counseling, screening for hepatitis C, educating women on engaging in newborn care, and care coordination with warm hand-offs.[49] In a pilot by the Northern New England Perinatal Quality Improvement Network (NNEPQIN), 8 hospitals integrated a perinatal clinical care checklist for women with OUD over 13 months in 2017 and 2018. Using collaborative improvement methods, participating hospitals incorporated the checklist in 78% of medical records, and they significantly increased access to naloxone (11% to 36%) and breastfeeding counseling (51% to 72%) for women with OUD. These early improvements highlighted the feasibility of a PQC to improve clinical care for women with OUD.[50]

The ILPQC Mothers and Newborns Affected by Opioids (MNO) initiative launched in May 2018 and is currently in progress, with 101 participating hospitals implementing ACOG guidelines with QI tools developed by ILPQC, including protocols, clinical care algorithms, and checklists for patients with OUD; provider and patient education materials; and case review and debrief with the clinical team for every patient with OUD.[51] MNO folders are being used as a QI strategy and have algorithms, checklists, provider counseling scripts, and patient education materials available in prenatal sites and delivery locations whenever a patient with OUD is identified. In May 2019, 1 year after implementation, hospitals reported that women screened with validated screening tools for substance use disorder on labor and delivery increased from 2% at baseline to 52%.[52] The percentage of hospitals with greater than or equal to 70% of women with OUD on MAT at delivery increased from 41% to 55% and the percentage of hospitals with greater than or equal to 70% of women with OUD linked to recovery services at delivery increased from 15% to 41%.[52] These early improvements show that a statewide collaborative can support hospital efforts to improve care and outcomes for women with OUD.

Immediate postpartum long-acting reversible contraception

Improved access to immediate postpartum long-acting reversible contraception (IPLARC) in the immediate postpartum period reduces short-interval pregnancies.[53] In 2016, ACOG supported hospital implementation of IPLARC as an effective contraception option for women and an opportunity to reduce barriers to postpartum contraception access.[54] PQCs launched initiatives to help hospitals to offer IPLARC, and many state public insurers have now unbundled billing of IPLARC placement from delivery. The South Carolina Birth Outcomes Initiative (SCBOI) launched an initiative to support hospital implementation of IPLARC and found, through review of Medicaid data charges, that 17% of Medicaid patients chose IPLARC during their delivery admission.[55] The Tennessee Initiative for Perinatal Quality (TIPQC) IPLARC initiative launched in 2018. Five of the 6 hospitals participating in the initiative were offering IPLARC after 1 year and provided 2012 LARC devices to women who chose IPLARC.[56] The ILPQC IPLARC initiative launched a first wave in May 2018 with 13 hospitals; only 3 were offering IPLARC at baseline and all 13 were providing IPLARC with all key components implemented by August 2019. ILPQC launched a second wave in May 2019, with 14 hospitals working to provide access to IPLARC by May 2020. To date, hospitals providing access to IPLARC cover nearly 40% of Illinois deliveries, with 5% of patients choosing IPLARC and 1907 women benefiting from improved access by receiving IPLARC.[57] PQCs have worked closely with state Medicaid and private insurers to address reimbursement issues and increase access to IPLARC as an available contraception option.

Emerging initiatives to address maternal morbidity and mortality

PQCs are developing other initiatives to address maternal morbidity and mortality. More than half of maternal deaths occur in the postpartum period and the recent ACOG guidelines on the fourth trimester have renewed focus on optimizing postpartum care.[30,58] ILPQC has recently launched an Improving Postpartum Access to Care (IPAC) initiative with 17 hospitals to implement universal early postpartum visits and standardize postpartum safety education, including signs and symptoms for when to seek care, benefits of an early maternal health safety check, and healthy pregnancy spacing.[57] Cardiovascular conditions are a leading cause of maternal death, with up to 68% deemed preventable.[30,59] CMQCC recently developed an Improving Health Care Response to Cardiovascular Disease in Pregnancy and Postpartum toolkit with some early validation tests of the cardiovascular disease algorithm in a birthing hospital.[60,61] Obstetric venous thromboembolism is another leading cause of SMM and mortality amenable to prevention, with a CMQCC toolkit available.[30,62]

Maternity Care Impact on Birth and Preterm Birth

The infant mortality was 5.79 per 1000 births in 2017.[63] Preterm birth is a leading cause of infant mortality.[64] Many PQCs initially formed as a strategy to reduce prematurity, and much of their early and current work focused on initiatives to reduce preterm birth and improve preterm birth outcomes. Initiatives focused on birth and preterm birth include reducing early elective deliveries before 39 weeks, increasing corticosteroid administration for eligible women, increasing progesterone administration to reduce preterm births, and optimizing breastfeeding.

Reducing elective delivery before 39 weeks

Elective, or non–medically indicated, deliveries before 39 weeks (also referred to as EED [early elective deliveries]) are associated with unnecessary neonatal morbidity and adverse long-term outcomes.[65,66] The March of Dimes (MOD) California Chapter worked with CMQCC to develop a toolkit to support hospital implementation of ACOG guidelines to reduce EED.[67,68] The MOD formed the Big 5 State Perinatal Collaborative with PQC and other state leaders in California, Florida, Illinois, New York, and Texas to implement the toolkit in 25 hospitals from September 2010 to February 2012. Participating hospitals reduced EED from 27.8% to 4.8% in 1 year.[69]

Other PQCs also launched initiatives to help hospitals reduce EED. The Ohio Perinatal Quality Collaborative (OPQC) 39-Weeks Delivery Charter Project launched in September 2008 with 20 hospitals and decreased EED from 25% in July 2008 to less than 5% by August 2009.[70,71] The Perinatal Quality Collaborative of North Carolina (PQCNC) 39 Weeks Project launched in 2009 with 33 hospitals. By the end of the project in 2010, EED before 39 weeks decreased from 2% to 1.1%, and the proportion of EED among all scheduled early-term deliveries decreased from 23.63% to 16.19%.[72] The New York State Perinatal Quality Collaborative (NYSPQC) Obstetrical Improvement Project to reduce non–medically indicated deliveries launched in 2012 with 96 hospitals.[73] Non–medically indicated delivery rates decreased among 17 regional perinatal centers in phase 1 from 24.8% in September 2010 to 6.7% by the start of phase 2 (June 2012) and 0.6% by the project end (November 2014).[74] This early PQC work on EED showed the value of the collaborative infrastructure.

Increasing antenatal corticosteroid administration for eligible women

Corticosteroid administration before anticipated preterm birth is associated with decreased neonatal morbidity and mortality, including lower severity and frequency of respiratory distress syndrome, necrotizing enterocolitis, and death.[75] The MOD Big 5 State Perinatal Collaborative Antenatal Corticosteroid Initiative in California, Florida, Illinois, New York, and Texas launched in January 2016 to develop resources to help 39 participating hospitals improve standardized identification of eligible patients and timely administration of antenatal corticosteroids (ACT).[76] By the end of the initiative in February 2017, participating hospitals reported a significant increase in use of a standard process for identification of eligible patients (59% to 88% of hospitals) and reduction in barriers to ACT administration, including standardized protocol (24% to 60%), uniform use (38% to 59%), and systems to track administration (38% to 59%).[76]

The California Perinatal Quality Care Collaborative (CPQCC) project on ACT administration, launched in 1999 with 25 hospitals, found an increased rate in ACT administration from 76% in 1998 to 86% in 2001.[77] Higher rates of ACT administration were sustained among participating hospitals compared with nonparticipating hospitals (85% vs 69%).[78] The OPQC Antenatal Corticosteroids Initiative launched in October 2011 with 18 hospitals and found high ACT administration rates over the course of the initiative (91.8%), achieving and maintaining the 90% goal by the second month of the initiative.[79] Hospital teams reported that a high-reliability culture and process, interdisciplinary engagement, and awareness of the evidence of the benefits of ACT contributed to their successful implementation of ACT.[80]

Progesterone to reduce premature births

The use of progesterone among women at risk for preterm birth can reduce the incidence of preterm birth.[81] The OPQC Progesterone Project launched in 2014 with 23 hospitals to support implementation of ACOG guidelines and decreased births before 32 weeks' gestation by 8.0% in participating hospitals compared with by 6.6% in all hospitals in the state. There was a 13% decrease in births before 32 weeks' gestation to women with prior preterm birth.[82,83]

Optimizing breastfeeding

ACOG provides guidelines for clinical management of breastfeeding to provide education, including information on improved maternal and infant health outcomes associated with breastfeeding, as well as support for breastfeeding.[84,85] The PQCNC Human Milk and Breastfeeding Initiative launched in late 2010 to support (1) newborn critical care center efforts to supply mother's milk to newborns less than 1500 g, and (2) maternity care center efforts to increase exclusive breastfeeding for term infants. Participating hospitals reported increased breastfeeding support by 425%, increased skin-to-skin contact days by 450%, and a 34% increase in exclusive breastfeeding rates through 28 days by January 2013.[86] The TIPQC Breastfeeding Promotion: Delivery and Postpartum initiative launched in 2012 with 11 hospitals. By 2013, they increased the aggregate Joint Commission Perinatal Care Performance Measure (PC)-05 measure of exclusive breast milk feeding from 37% to 42%. Wave 2 launched in 2014 with additional hospitals for a total of 18 hospital teams achieving improvement in aggregate Joint Commission PC-05 rates from 40.9% to 44.8% by the end of 2015.[87]

Birth Equity

The burden of maternal and infant morbidity and mortality in the United States is disproportionately borne by African Americans. African American women are 3 times as likely as white women to die in pregnancy through 1 year postpartum from a pregnancy-related cause,[4] and are more likely to deliver an infant preterm: 14% compared with 9% for non-Hispanic white women.[88] There is also a 12% difference in the rate of breastfeeding initiation between non-Hispanic black and white women in the United States.[27] PQCs are working to address these disparities across initiatives and are exploring ways to develop targeted initiatives on birth equity, including resources from the recent AIM Reduction of Peripartum Racial/Ethnic Disparities bundle.[89] In 2018, the CMQCC launched the California Birth Equity Collaborative, starting with a pilot initiative working with 5 hospitals and community stakeholders to develop and test key resources to support hospital system and culture change to promote birth equity, including a patient-reported experience metric, online educational resources, and best-practice interventions.[90] Other PQCs are working to develop key strategies for promoting birth equity, including providing respectful care; addressing social determinants of health; engaging patients, communities, and birth partners; and engaging and educating providers with incorporation of implicit bias training.

SUMMARY

The goal of PQCs is to partner with hospitals, providers, nurses, patients, public health, and other stakeholders, using QI strategies to implement evidence-based practices to improve outcomes for mothers and newborns.[5] As states across the country develop and expand PQCs, it is important to consider strategies to increase the capacity of PQCs to succeed.[15]

It must be recognized that PQCs are at varying levels of development. Although most states have an identified PQC organization, many PQCs currently lack the personnel and infrastructure to function optimally. Thus, many have yet to reach their maximum potential to make measurable improvements in statewide maternal and infant care and outcomes. Although many PQCs are clearly making a difference to address the current challenges in maternal and newborn health, significant work remains to get every PQC to the level where they can make sustainable and significant population-level improvements in maternal health outcomes.

Progress in PQC development, sustainability, and impact on maternal outcomes depends on several key factors. PQC development and sustainability are built on adequate staffing and infrastructure. Progress also depends on the involvement of critical stakeholders and champions to provide leadership for effective QI initiatives, and the optimal engagement of clinical teams to achieve sustainable improvements in care. In addition, key partnerships at the state and federal levels can help to address maternal morbidity and mortality, including (1) ongoing collaborations with AIM on implementation of maternal safety bundles, which are a key resources for QI initiatives; (2) expanding ties at the state level with maternal mortality review committees and departments of public health to promote implementation of maternal mortality prevention strategies and efforts to address birth equity; and (3) ongoing support at the national and state levels from key stakeholders (eg, national obstetric and nursing organizations, hospital associations, maternal health partners, and payers). The NNPQC, supported by the CDC and coordinated by NICHQ, is another important resource for ongoing technical support for PQCs, creating opportunities for collaborative learning between early and more developed PQCs.

PQCs can make a difference and improve a range of outcomes. Given the urgent challenges facing maternal and newborn health across the country, there is a clear need for additional efforts to develop and sustain PQCs nationwide. PQCs can be well positioned to achieve the goal of sustainable improvements in maternal and newborn care and outcomes.

DISCLOSURE

The authors disclose no commercial or financial conflicts of interest. ILPQC, Dr A.E.B. Borders, principal investigator, is funded by the Centers for Disease Control and Prevention, Illinois Department of Public Health, Illinois Department of Human Services, University of Illinois at Chicago, Pritzker Family Foundation, and the Alliance for Innovation on Maternal Health.

Best Practices

What is the current practice? State-based perinatal quality collaboratives

State-based PQCs have shown that the application of collaborative improvement science methods can lead to better perinatal health outcomes by:
- Advancing evidence-informed clinical practices and processes using QI strategies.
- Addressing gaps by implementing statewide initiatives working with clinical teams, obstetric provider and nursing leaders, patients and families, public health officials, and other stakeholders to spread best practices, reduce variation in practice, reduce health care inequities, and optimize efforts to improve perinatal care and outcomes.

What changes in current practice are likely to improve outcomes?

- Use of the collaborative learning model to share knowledge and experiences among clinical teams working toward unified objectives for improvement.

- Use of rapid-response data by clinical teams to track and compare progress toward meeting those objectives.
- Provision of QI science support and assistance to clinical teams.
- Engage obstetric provider champions at the state, hospital, and clinical levels to promote buy-in and achieve clinical culture change.

Major recommendations

- Given the urgent challenges facing maternal and newborn health across the country, an emphasis on developing and sustaining PQCs nationwide is needed.
- Physician, nursing, and public health champions provide leadership for effective QI initiatives, optimally engage hospital teams, and achieve sustainable improvements in care.
- Key partnerships can be promoted with state and federal efforts to address maternal morbidity and mortality to ensure effective collaboration.

Summary sentence

- PQCs in many states are an effective intervention to improve maternal health outcomes. With appropriate staffing, infrastructure, and partnerships, PQCs can be well positioned to achieve the goal of sustainable improvements in maternal and newborn care and outcomes nationwide.

REFERENCES

1. Hoyert DL, Minino AM. Maternal mortality in the United States: changes in coding, publication, and data release, 2018. Natl Vital Stat Rep 2020;69:1–18. Available at: https://www.cdc.gov/nchs/data/nvsr/nvsr69/nvsr69_02-508.pdf. Accessed January 30, 2020.
2. Ely DM, Driscoll AK. Infant mortality in the United States, 2017: data from the period linked birth/infant death file. Natl Vital Stat Rep 2019;68(10):1–20. Available at: https://www.cdc.gov/nchs/data/nvsr/nvsr68/nvsr68_10-508.pdf. Accessed August 1, 2019.
3. Organization for Economic Co-operation and Development. Infant mortality rates. 2020. Available at: https://data.oecd.org/healthstat/infant-mortality-rates.htm.
4. Petersen EE, Davis NL, Goodman D, et al. Racial/ethnic disparities in pregnancy-related deaths - United States, 2007–2016. MMWR Morb Mortal Wkly Rep 2019; 68(35):762–5. Available at: https://www.cdc.gov/mmwr/volumes/68/wr/mm6835a3.htm.
5. Henderson ZT, Ernst K, Simpson KR, et al. The National Network of State Perinatal Quality Collaboratives: a growing movement to improve maternal and infant health. J Womens Health 2018;27(2):123.
6. Gould JB. The role of regional collaboratives: the California Perinatal Quality Care Collaborative model. Clin Perinatol 2010;37(1):71–86.
7. Centers for Disease Control and Prevention. State perinatal quality collaboratives. 2020. Available at: https://www.cdc.gov/reproductivehealth/maternalinfanthealth/pqc-states.html. Accessed March 5, 2020.
8. Institute of Medicine (US) Committee on Quality of Health Care in America. To err is human: building a safer health system. 2001. Available at: https://www.nap.edu/catalog/9728/to-err-is-human-building-a-safer-health-system.
9. Institute of Medicine (US) Committee on Quality of Health Care in America. Crossing the quality chasm: a new health system for the 21st century. 2001. Available at: https://www.nap.edu/catalog/25152/crossing-the-global-quality-chasm-improving-health-care-worldwide.

10. Abraham MR, Ashton DM, Badura MB, et al. Toward improving the outcome of pregnancy III: enhancing perinatal health through quality, safety and performance initiatives. 2010. Available at: http://www.marchofdimes.org/materials/toward-improving-the-outcome-of-pregnancy-iii.pdf.

11. The Joint Commission. Provision of care, treatment, and services standards for maternal safety. *R3 Report: Requirement, Rationale, Reference*. 2019(R3). Available at: https://www.jointcommission.org/-/media/tjc/documents/standards/r3-reports/r3_24_maternal_safety_hap_9_6_19_final1.pdf. Accessed August 21, 2019.

12. Mahoney J. The Alliance for Innovation in Maternal Health Care: a way forward. Clin Obstet Gynecol 2018;61(2):400–10.

13. Institute for Healthcare Improvement. The breakthrough series: IHI's collaborative model for achieving breakthrough improvement. Innovation Series White Paper. 2003. Available at: http://www.ihi.org/resources/Pages/IHIWhitePapers/TheBreakthroughSeriesIHIsCollaborativeModelforAchievingBreakthroughImprovement.aspx.

14. Centers for Disease Control and Prevention. Developing and sustaining perinatal quality collaboratives - a resource guide for states. 2016. Available at: https://www.cdc.gov/reproductivehealth/maternalinfanthealth/pdf/Best-Practices-for-Developing-and-Sustaining-Perinatal-Quality-Collaboratives_tagged508.pdf.

15. Lee King PA, Young D, Borders AEB. A framework to harness the power of quality collaboratives to improve perinatal outcomes. Clin Obstet Gynecol 2019;62(3):606.

16. Mehta PK, Kieltyka L, Bachhuber MA, et al. Racial inequities in preventable pregnancy-related deaths in Louisiana, 2011-2016. Obstet Gynecol 2020;135(2):276.

17. Goodman DA; Centers for Disease Control and Prevention. Safe motherhood: an update from CDC. Presented at the Title V Technical Assistance Meeting. Arlington, VA. October 15, 2018.

18. D'Alton ME, Bonanno CA, Berkowitz RL, et al. Putting the "M" back in maternal-fetal medicine. Am J Obstet Gynecol 2013;208(6):442.

19. Clark SL, Belfort MA, Dildy GA, et al. Maternal death in the 21st century: causes, prevention, and relationship to cesarean delivery. Am J Obstet Gynecol 2008;199(1):36.e1–5.

20. The Joint Commission. Specifications manual for Joint Commission national quality core measures (2019A); perinatal care. 2019. Available at: https://manual.jointcommission.org/releases/TJC2019A/PerinatalCare.html. Accessed February 7, 2020.

21. Healthy People. MICH-7.1 Reduce cesarean births among low-risk women with no prior births. 2019. Available at: https://www.healthypeople.gov/node/4900/data_details#revision_history_header. Accessed February 9, 2020.

22. American College of Obstetricians and Gynecologists, Society for Maternal-Fetal Medicine. Obstetric care consensus no. 1: safe prevention of the primary cesarean delivery. Obstet Gynecol 2014;123:693–711.

23. Lagrew DC, Low LK, Brennan R, et al. National partnership for maternal safety: consensus bundle on safe reduction of primary cesarean births-supporting intended vaginal births. Obstet Gynecol 2018;131(3):503–13.

24. Smith H, Peterson N, Lagrew D, et al. Toolkit to support vaginal birth and reduce primary cesareans. 2017. Available at: https://www.cmqcc.org/VBirthToolkitResource. Accessed February 9, 2020.

25. Lagrew DC, Mills M, Mikes K, et al. 822: rapid reduction of the NTSV CS rate in multiple community hospitals using a multi-dimensional QI approach. Am J Obstet Gynecol 2017;216(1):S471–2.

26. Main EK, Chang S-C, Cape V, et al. Safety assessment of a large-scale improvement collaborative to reduce nulliparous cesarean delivery rates. Obstet Gynecol 2019;133(4):613.

27. Centers for Disease Control and Prevention. National Center for Chronic Disease Prevention and Health Promotion, Division of Nutrition, Physical Activity, and Obesity. Data, Trend and Maps [online]. Available at: https://www.cdc.gov/nccdphp/dnpao/data-trends-maps/index.html. Accessed May 18, 2020.

28. Florida Perinatal Quality Collaborative. Promoting primary vaginal deliveries initiative, Provide 2.0: the next generation. 2019. Available at: https://health.usf.edu/-/media/Files/Public-Health/Chiles-Center/FPQC/PROVIDEWebinar-PROVIDE2-May2019.ashx?la=en&hash=60D6DEC3C9205DB38333C58516424A8C627A06AA. Accessed February 9, 2020.

29. Bronson EA. "Always PROVIDE": 76 Florida hospitals commit to promote primary vaginal deliveries. 2019. Available at: https://hscweb3.hsc.usf.edu/health/publichealth/news/always-provide-76-florida-hospitals-commit-to-promote-primary-vaginal-deliveries/.

30. Petersen EE, Davis NL, Goodman D, et al. Vital signs: pregnancy-related deaths, United States, 2011-2015, and strategies for prevention, 13 states, 2013-2017. MMWR Morb Mortal Wkly Rep 2019;68:423–9. Available at: https://www.cdc.gov/vitalsigns/maternal-deaths/.

31. Main EK, McCain CL, Morton CH, et al. Pregnancy-related mortality in California: causes, characteristics, and improvement opportunities. Obstet Gynecol 2015;125(4):938.

32. Shields LE. Practice bulletin No. 183 summary: postpartum hemorrhage. Obstet Gynecol 2017;130(4):923–5.

33. Main EK, Goffman D, Scavone BM, et al. National partnership for maternal safety: consensus bundle on obstetric hemorrhage. J Obstet Gynecol Neonatal Nurs 2015;44(4):462–70.

34. Burgansky A, Montalto D, Siddiqui NA. The safe motherhood initiative: the development and implementation of standardized obstetric care bundles in New York. Semin Perinatol 2016;40(2):124–31.

35. Florida Perinatal Quality Collaborative. Obstetric hemorrhage initiative toolkit. 2014. Available at: https://health.usf.edu/publichealth/chiles/fpqc/OHI. Accessed February 9, 2020.

36. Lyndon A, Lagrew D, Shields L, et al. Improving health care response to obstetric hemorrhage version 2.0: a California quality improvement toolkit. 2015. Available at: https://www.cmqcc.org/resources-tool-kits/toolkits/ob-hemorrhage-toolkit. Accessed February 9, 2020.

37. Florida Perinatal Quality Collaborative. Obstetric hemorrhage initiative final data report. 2015. Available at: https://health.usf.edu/-/media/Files/Public-Health/Chiles-Center/FPQC/FinalOHIDataReport.ashx?la=en&hash=F2E3E479F5FA7AFFFD4EE3D3C3CBCDDE737CFE00.

38. Vamos CA, Cantor A, Thompson EL, et al. The obstetric hemorrhage initiative (OHI) in Florida: the role of intervention characteristics in influencing implementation experiences among multidisciplinary hospital staff. Matern Child Health J 2016;20(10):2003.

39. Main EK, Cape V, Abreo A, et al. Reduction of severe maternal morbidity from hemorrhage using a state perinatal quality collaborative. Am J Obstet Gynecol 2017;216(3):298.e1.

40. American College of Obstetricians and Gynecologists. Emergent therapy for acute-onset, severe hypertension during pregnancy and the postpartum period. ACOG committee opinion no. 767. Obstet Gynecol 2019;133:e174–80.

41. Bernstein PS, Martin JN, Barton JR, et al. Consensus bundle on severe hypertension during pregnancy and the postpartum period. J Midwifery Womens Health 2017;62(4):493.

42. Shields L, Kilpatrick S, Melsop K, et al. 103: timely assessment and treatment of preeclampsia reduces maternal morbidity. Am J Obstet Gynecol 2015; 212(1):S69.

43. California Maternal Quality Care Collaborative. Preeclampsia collaboratives. 2020. Available at: https://www.cmqcc.org/qi-initiatives/preeclampsia/preeclampsia-collaboratives. Accessed February 9, 2020.

44. Lee King P, Keenan-Devlin L, Gordon C, et al. 4: reducing time to treatment for severe maternal hypertension through statewide quality improvement. Am J Obstet Gynecol 2018;218(1):S4.

45. Gavigan S, Rosenbergy N, Hurlbert J. Proactively preventing maternal hemorrhage-related deaths. *Leading Hospital Improvement*. 2019. Available at: https://www.jointcommission.org/en/resources/news-and-multimedia/blogs/leading-hospital-improvement/2019/11/proactively-preventing-maternal-hemorrhagerelated-deaths/. Accessed February 20, 2020.

46. Haight S, Ko J, Tong VT, et al. Opioid use disorder documented at delivery hospitalization — United States, 1999–2014. MMWR Morb Mortal Wkly Rep 2018; 67(31):845–9.

47. deaths. BUSctrapm. Report from nine maternal mortality review committees. 2018. Available at: https://www.cdcfoundation.org/sites/default/files/files/ReportfromNineMMRCs.pdf.

48. American College of Obstetricians and Gynecologists. Opioid use and opioid use disorder in pregnancy. committee opinion no. 711. Obstet Gynecol 2017;130: e81–94.

49. Krans EE, Campopiano M, Cleveland LM, et al. National partnership for maternal safety: consensus bundle on obstetric care for women with opioid use disorder. Obstet Gynecol 2019;134(2):365.

50. Goodman D, Zagaria A, Flanagan V, et al. Feasibility and acceptability of a checklist and learning collaborative to promote quality and safety in the perinatal care of women with opioid use disorders. J Midwifery Womens Health 2019;64(1): 104–11.

51. Illinois Perinatal Quality Collaborative. Mothers and newborns affected by opioids - OB. 2018. Available at: https://ilpqc.org/mothers-and-newborns-affected-by-opioids-ob-initiative/. Accessed February 9, 2020.

52. Borders A, Lee King P, Weiss D, et al. 160: improving outcomes for mothers affected by opioids through statewide quality improvement. Am J Obstet Gynecol 2020;222(1):S116.

53. Kroelinger CDMI, DeSisto CL, Estrich C, et al. State-identified implementation strategies to increase uptake of immediate postpartum long-acting reversible contraception policies. J Womens Health 2018;28(3):346–56.

54. American College of Obstetricians and Gynecologists. Immediate postpartum long-acting reversible contraception. Obstet Gynecol 2016;128:e32–7.

55. Association of State and Territorial Health Officials. South Carolina increases access to LARCs immediately postpartum to reduce unintended pregnancy. 2017. Available at: https://www.astho.org/Maternal-and-Child-Health/South-Carolina-Increases-Access-to-LARCs-Immediately-Postpartum-to-Reduce-Unintended-Pregnancy/.

56. Lacy MM, McMurtry Baird S, Scott TA, et al. Statewide quality improvement initiative to implement immediate postpartum long-acting reversible contraception. Am J Obstet Gynecol 2020;222(4, Supplement):S910.e1–8.

57. Illinois Perinatal Quality Collaborative. ILPQC stronger together: 2019 review and onward to 2020. 2019. Available at: https://ilpqc.org/ILPQC%202020%2B/Annual%20Conferences/2019%20Annual%20Conference/1_Borders%20et%20al_ILPQC%20A%20Year%20in%20Review_%28Grand%20Ballroom%20A-F%29_ALL%20FINAL_11.1.2019.pdf. Accessed March 10, 2020.

58. American College of Obstetricians and Gynecologists. Optimizing postpartum care. ACOG committee opinion no. 736. Obstet Gynecol 2018;131:e140–50.

59. Hameed AB, Lawton ES, McCain CL, et al. Pregnancy-related cardiovascular deaths in California: beyond peripartum cardiomyopathy. Am J Obstet Gynecol 2015;213(3):379.e1–10.

60. Hameed AB, Morton CH, Moore A. Improving health care response to cardiovascular disease in pregnancy and postpartum. 2017. Available at: https://www.cmqcc.org/resources-toolkits/toolkits/improving-health-care-response-cardiovascular-disease-pregnancy-and.

61. Crosland BA, Blumenthal EA, Senderoff DS, et al. 833: heart of the matter: preliminary-analysis of the California maternal quality care collaborative cardiovascular disease toolkit. Am J Obstet Gynecol 2019;220(1):S544.

62. Hameed AB, Friedman A, Peterson N, et al. Improving health care response to maternal venous thromboembolism. 2018. Available at: https://www.cmqcc.org/resources-toolkits/toolkits/improving-health-care-response-maternal-venous-thromboembolism.

63. Centers for Disease Control and Prevention. Infant mortality. 2019. Available at: https://www.cdc.gov/reproductivehealth/maternalinfanthealth/infantmortality.htm#causes. Accessed January 30, 2020.

64. Kochanek KDM SL, Xu J, Arias E. Deaths: final data for 2017. Natl Vital Stat Rep 2019;68(9):1–77. Available at: https://www.cdc.gov/nchs/data/nvsr/nvsr68/nvsr68_09-508.pdf. Accessed June 24, 2019.

65. Clark SL, Miller DD, Belfort MA, et al. Neonatal and maternal outcomes associated with elective term delivery. Am J Obstet Gynecol 2009;200(2):156.e1–4.

66. Noble KG, Fifer WP, Rauh VA, et al. Academic achievement varies with gestational age among children born at term. Pediatrics 2012;130(2):E257.

67. Main E, Oshiro B, Chagolla B, et al. Elimination of non-medically indicated (elective) deliveries before 39 weeks gestational age. 2010. Available at: https://www.marchofdimes.org/professionals/less-than-39-weeks-toolkit.aspx.

68. American College of Obstetricians and Gynecologists. Avoidance of nonmedically indicated early-term deliveries and associated neonatal morbidities. ACOG committee opinion no. 765. Obstet Gynecol 2019;133:e156–63.

69. Oshiro BT, Kowalewski L, Sappenfield W, et al. A multistate quality improvement program to decrease elective deliveries before 39 weeks of gestation. Obstet Gynecol 2013;121(5):1025.

70. Donovan EF, Lannon C, Bailit J, et al. A statewide initiative to reduce inappropriate scheduled births at 36 0/7–38 6/7 weeks' gestation. Am J Obstet Gynecol 2010;202(3):243.e1–8.

71. Bailit JL, Iams J, Silber A, et al. Changes in the indications for scheduled births to reduce nonmedically indicated deliveries occurring before 39 weeks of gestation. Obstet Gynecol 2012;120(2 Pt 1):241.

72. Berrien K, Devente J, French A, et al. The perinatal quality collaborative of North Carolina's 39 weeks project: a quality improvement program to decrease elective deliveries before 39 weeks of gestation. N C Med J 2014;75(3):169–76.

73. Perinatal quality collaborative success story: New York State Perinatal Quality Collaborative increases the proportion of babies born full-term. 2014. Available at: https://www.albany.edu/cphce/nyspqcpublic/success_stories_8-2014.pdf.

74. Kacica M, Glantz J, Xiong K, et al. A statewide quality improvement initiative to reduce non-medically indicated scheduled deliveries. Matern Child Health J 2017;21(4):932–41.

75. Crowley P. Prophylactic corticosteroids for preterm birth. Cochrane Database Syst Rev 2000;(2):CD000065.

76. March of Dimes. Optimize the administration of antenatal corticosteroids (ACS) for impending preterm births – update. 2019. Available at: https://patientsafetymovement.org/commitments/optimize-the-administration-of-antenatal-corticosteroids-acs-for-impending-preterm-births-update-06-24-19/.

77. Wirtschafter DD, Danielsen BH, Main EK, et al. Promoting antenatal steroid use for fetal maturation: results from the California Perinatal Quality Care Collaborative. J Pediatr 2006;148(5):606–12.e1.

78. Lee HC, Lyndon A, Blumenfeld YJ, et al. Antenatal steroid administration for premature neonates in California. Obstet Gynecol 2011;117(3):603–9.

79. Ohio Perinatal Quality Collaborative Writing Committee. A statewide project to promote optimal use of antenatal corticosteroids (ANCS). Am J Obstet Gynecol 2013;208(1):S224.

80. Kaplan HC, Sherman SN, Cleveland C, et al. Reliable implementation of evidence: a qualitative study of antenatal corticosteroid administration in Ohio hospitals. BMJ Qual Saf 2016;25(3):173.

81. Hassan SS, Romero R, Vidyadhari D, et al. Vaginal progesterone reduces the rate of preterm birth in women with a sonographic short cervix: a multicenter, randomized, double-blind, placebo-controlled trial. Ultrasound Obstet Gynecol 2011;38(1):18–31.

82. Iams JD, Applegate MS, Marcotte MP, et al. A state wide progestogen promotion program in Ohio. Obstet Gynecol 2017;129(2):337–46.

83. American College of Obstetricians and Gynecologists. Prediction and prevention of preterm birth. practice bulletin no. 130. Obstet Gynecol 2012;120:964–73.

84. American College of Obstetricians and Gynecologists. Optimizing support for breastfeeding as part of obstetric practice. ACOG committee opinion no. 756. Obstet Gynecol 2018;132:e187–96.

85. Section on Breastfeeding. Breastfeeding and the use of human milk. Pediatrics 2012;129(3):e827.

86. Perinatal Quality Collaborative North Carolina. Human milk and breastfeeding: increasing exclusivity in the hospital. 2013. Available at: https://www.pqcnc.org/initiatives/milk-nccc. Accessed February 9, 2020.

87. Tennessee Initiative for Perinatal Quality Care. Breastfeeding promotion: delivery and postpartum. 2016. Available at: https://tipqc.org/breastfeeding-promotion/. Accessed February 9, 2020.

88. Martin JA, Hamilton BE, Osterman MJK. Births in the United States, 2018. NCHS Data Brief 2019;(346):1–8. Available at: https://www.cdc.gov/nchs/data/databriefs/db346-h.pdf.

89. Howell EA, Brown H, Brumley J, et al. Reduction of peripartum racial and ethnic disparities: a conceptual framework and maternal safety consensus bundle. Obstet Gynecol 2018;131(5):770.
90. California Maternal Quality Care Collaborative. Birth equity: California birth equity collaborative: improving care, experiences and outcomes for black mothers. 2019. Available at: https://www.cmqcc.org/qi-initiatives/birth-equity. Accessed March 3, 2020.

Optimizing Term Delivery and Mode of Delivery

Timothy Wen, MD, MPH[a], Amy L. Turitz, MD[b],*

KEYWORDS

- Full-term delivery • Early term delivery • Obstetric comorbidities • Mode of delivery

KEY POINTS

- Nonindicated deliveries are recommended to occur no earlier than 39 weeks and 0 days to optimize neonatal outcomes.
- There are medical, obstetric, and fetal indications that may necessitate late preterm or early term delivery given the pathophysiology of certain conditions.
- Maternal medical and obstetric indications for early term delivery are principled according to the risk they pose to maternal and fetal health with prolongation of pregnancy.
- Fetal indications for early term delivery are predicated on the principle of balancing the risk of intrauterine stillbirth with expectant management to the risk of postnatal morbidity and mortality with early delivery.
- As maternal comorbidities and obstetric complications increase in the United States, further research is needed to provide evidence-based recommendations for the optimal timing of delivery for each condition.

INTRODUCTION

Early term deliveries are defined as occurring between 37 weeks 0 days and 38 weeks 6 days, and full-term deliveries are defined as occurring between 39 weeks and 0 days and 40 weeks and 6 days.[1] Neonates born before 37 weeks are classified as preterm and those after 41 weeks as late-term (between 41 weeks 0 days to 41 weeks 6 days) or postterm (42 weeks 0 days and beyond).[1,2] Both preterm and late/postterm deliveries are associated with their own set of risks and adverse neonatal outcomes.[2] In the past, it was assumed that neonatal outcomes of term deliveries were optimized and uniform. More recently, a growing body of evidence has demonstrated disparities in outcomes when stratified by week of gestation during the term period.[3] Tita and colleagues[4] (2009) noted that in more than one-third of nonmedically indicated Cesarean

a Division of Maternal Fetal Medicine, Department of Obstetrics, Gynecology and Reproductive Sciences, University of California, San Francisco, CA 94158, USA; b Division of Maternal Fetal Medicine, Department of Obstetrics and Gynecology, Columbia University Irving Medical Center, 622 West 168th Street, New York, NY 10032, USA
* Corresponding author.
E-mail address: alt2153@cumc.columbia.edu

Clin Perinatol 47 (2020) 799–815
https://doi.org/10.1016/j.clp.2020.08.010
0095-5108/20/© 2020 Elsevier Inc. All rights reserved.

deliveries performed in the early term period, neonates were at increased risk for significant complications compared with their counterparts born at 39 week and beyond. Subsequent studies in both the neonatal and obstetric literature have highlighted worse outcomes for early term deliveries. As a result, the March of Dimes and *Eunice Kennedy Shriver* National Institute for Child Health and Human Development have championed the notion of preventing unnecessary early term births.[5,6] In general, proposed criteria for low-risk term deliveries are recommended to occur no earlier than 39 weeks, whereas timing of indicated deliveries remains a more nebulous concept.

HISTORY

In 2008, the National Quality Foundation (NQF) organized a multidisciplinary body including representatives from maternal fetal medicine, obstetrics and gynecology, neonatology, midwifery, and nursing to develop a set of perinatal measures meant to increase the quality of maternal care and optimize neonatal outcomes.[7,8] One of the first quality measures to come out of this collaboration focused on optimizing the timing of term deliveries.[7] The increasing number of provider-driven deliveries coupled with the decreasing gestational age at birth motivated the development of the "39-week rule," restricting nonmedically indicated deliveries before 39 weeks.[4,7–9]

Since its inception, the "39-week rule" has been accepted by various organizations, such as the Society of Maternal Fetal Medicine and the American College of Obstetricians and Gynecologists, and progressively enforced through a combination of hospital policies and financial incentives.[7,10] Adherence to the clinical practice of the "39-week rule" has been the subject of multiple studies, which have not surprisingly demonstrated reductions in early term deliveries.[9,11–13] These studies have also documented improvement in neonatal outcomes such as respiratory distress syndrome, transient tachypnea of the newborn, hypoglycemia, and admissions to the neonatal intensive care unit (NICU).[11,14,15] In 2018, the "39-week rule" was codified among low-risk nulliparous women with the publication of the ARRIVE (A Randomized Trial of Induction Versus Expectant Management) trial with subsequent studies noting benefits among multiparous women as well.[16–18]

Although the NQF's perinatal guideline of the "39-week rule" applies to elective, nonmedically indicated deliveries, there exists an entire subset of medically indicated deliveries whose optimal timing may be less clear from the existing literature. Furthermore, although the clinical benefits of elective induction at or beyond 39 weeks are numerous, there are also critiques and criticisms, as rates of term stillbirths have not changed and economic costs have increased in the labor and delivery units since the publication of ARRIVE. In this review, the authors sought to assess the optimal timing of delivery within the term period in the context of various maternal, fetal, and obstetric conditions.

MATERNAL CONSIDERATIONS

Although the obstetric governing bodies have come to agreement with regard to induction of labor among low-risk women, American College of Obstetricians and Gynecologists (ACOG) does not recommend deferring delivery to the 39th week if there is a maternal condition necessitating earlier delivery.[19] Given the increasing clinical complexity of the obstetric population in the United States with the increase of obesity, chronic hypertension, diabetes, and increasing maternal age at delivery, optimal timing of delivery for maternal indications is of paramount importance.

Hypertension

Chronic hypertension

Chronic hypertension affects 1% to 5% of pregnancies and is expected to increase along with the rates of obesity and advancing maternal age in the obstetric population.[20,21] Controversy exists in the timing of delivery for pregnancies complicated by chronic hypertension, with the benefits of early term delivery including decreased risks of superimposed preeclampsia, placental abruption, and stillbirth.[22] Current recommendations are based on the degree of disease control. Those not on medications are recommended for delivery between 38 and 39 weeks, whereas those well controlled on medication are recommended for delivery between 37 and 39 weeks. For patients whose disease is not well controlled, delivery may be considered even earlier, between 36 and 37 weeks.[19] A recent study by Ram and colleagues[22] (2018) supports the recommendation for delivery in well-controlled patients with chronic hypertension at 38 or 39 weeks. In this study, induction at 38 or 39 weeks in women with chronic hypertension was associated with a lower risk of new-onset superimposed preeclampsia, eclampsia, and Cesarean delivery compared with expectantly managed chronic hypertensives.[22] A similar review by Chahine and Sibai (2019) supported stratifying women with hypertension as low or high risk based on comorbid conditions, medication usage, or other fetal conditions, and based on delivery timing on this delineation.[23]

Hypertensive diseases of pregnancy

Hypertensive diseases of pregnancy (HDP), including gestational hypertension and preeclampsia, affect 3% to 10% of all pregnancies and are significant causes of maternal and neonatal morbidity and mortality.[24–29] ACOG currently recommends delivery at 37 weeks for mild disease or at diagnosis beyond 37 weeks given the increasing risks of maternal and fetal complications.[19,30] In support of these recommendations, a recent meta-analysis by Bernardes and colleagues[31] (2019) of randomized controlled trials comparing immediate delivery with expectant management of women with gestational hypertension noted a higher risk of progression to HELLP syndrome and eclampsia among expectantly managed women.

Diabetes

Similar to chronic hypertension, timing of delivery of the diabetic patient depends on the degree of disease control. Although diabetic patients in general are at higher risk of fetal macrosomia, stillbirth, and HDP compared with nondiabetic patients, poor glucose control further exacerbates these risks. Balancing these risks against neonatal outcomes stratified by gestational age during the term period requires thoughtful consideration.

Patients with gestational diabetes (GDM) are subdivided into those requiring medical management and those who are controlled by diet and lifestyle changes.[32] In general, those who are nonmedically managed or medically managed with good control may be delivered later than their medically managed and/or poorly controlled counterparts.[19] This is supported by a retrospective cohort study by Rosenstein and colleagues (2012) in which women with gestational diabetes who were expectantly managed were compared with those who underwent planned delivery between 37 and 39 weeks. The study noted higher risk of perinatal mortality for expectantly managed pregnancies compared with those delivered at 39 weeks, supporting the idea of delivery at 39 weeks.[32,33] A decision analysis by Niu and colleagues[34] (2014) examining delivery timing ofs patients with GDM concluded that 38 weeks was the ideal time for delivery in order to balance the risks of diabetes and neonatal mortality and morbidity. When adjusting for the baseline stillbirth rate, these data could be extrapolated to suggest that delivery at 39 weeks for patients with well-controlled GDM is optimal.[32,34]

The recommendation for early term delivery for medically managed patients with GDM comes primarily from a prospective, randomized controlled trial by Kios (1993) comparing induction at 39 weeks to expectant management. Although the Cesarean delivery rate was not significantly different, the rates of large-for-gestational-age (LGA) infants and shoulder dystocia were significantly higher in the expectantly managed groups (23% vs 10% and 3% vs 0%, respectively).[35,36] Additional studies support induction at 38 weeks for insulin-dependent GDM patients, demonstrating fewer cases of shoulder dystocia compared with expectant management.[37]

Similar to GDM, the rationale for labor induction of women with pregestational diabetes mellitus (PGDM) is to prevent stillbirth, excessive fetal growth, and its associated complications.[38] Brown and colleagues[39] (2019) conducted a retrospective population registry study of women with PGDM comparing the risk of Cesarean delivery with induction at 38 weeks to expectant management up to 39 weeks and 0 days. They found that the risk of Cesarean delivery between the 2 groups was not different, although the 2 groups were convenience samples and there was a higher composite morbidity noted with the group induced at 38 weeks compared with the expectantly managed group.[39] Similar to GDM, timing of delivery of patients with PGDM is also based on glycemic control. Patients with poor control are typically recommended to deliver in the early term period to decrease risks of macrosomia, stillbirth, and other obstetric risks. The presence of preexisting diabetic-related comorbidities, such as vasculopathy, nephropathy, or retinopathy, are also further used to justify early term delivery.[32,40,41] Further large scale randomized controlled trials are needed to shed light on the optimal delivery timing of these patients.

Intrahepatic cholestasis of pregnancy

Intrahepatic cholestasis of pregnancy (ICP) is one of the most common hepatic disorders of pregnancy, characterized by pruritus and abnormal liver function in severe cases.[42] Although most women afflicted with ICP have no long-term hepatic sequelae, the risk of fetal complications, namely stillbirth, is higher with risks of mortality ranging up to 2%.[43–45] Elective early delivery of ICP has been the mainstay of management in these patients due to increasing rates of fetal demise with advancing gestational age, particularly after the 36th week.[46] A decision analysis done by Lo and colleagues[47] (2014) noted that delivery at 36 weeks was associated with a lower risk of stillbirth and maximized quality life adjusted years compared with delivery at 37 weeks, leading to the conclusion that the optimal time of delivery is at 36 weeks. This was further bolstered by Puljic and colleagues[48] (2015) who conducted a retrospective study of 1.6 million deliveries noting that the risk of perinatal mortality associated with delivery and stillbirth substantially shifted after 36 weeks. Studies have looked into using serum bile acids to inform delivery timing, as higher levels may be associated with a higher risk of stillbirth. Ovadia and colleagues[49] (2019) conducted a meta-analysis of 23 studies, demonstrating that elevated total bile acid concentrations greater than 100 umol/L were associated with 3.44% stillbirth prevalence after 24 weeks compared with the general population stillbirth rate of 0.3% to 0.4%, leading some to suggest that those with bile acid concentrations greater than 100umol/L should aim to be delivered between 35 and 36 weeks.[50] Currently, SMFM does not recommend using bile acids to inform delivery timing, and there are no current trials assessing optimal timing of delivery in this population.[51] ACOG currently recommends delivery at 36 to 37 weeks in light of the risks of stillbirth.[19]

Obesity

Obesity is defined as having a body mass index (BMI) of 30 kg/meters^2 or greater and is a condition of increasing prevalence in the United States and among the obstetric population. Obese patients are more likely to have pre-existing comorbidities such as diabetes and chronic hypertension and are also at increased risk of pregnancy-specific complications including HDP, Cesarean delivery, and stillbirth. Rates of stillbirth increase proportionally with BMI with odds ratios of 5.04 of stillbirth in women with a BMI higher than 50.[52] Similarly, multiple studies have noted a linear relationship between increasing BMI and the risk for Cesarean delivery.[53,54] In a large retrospective Consortium on Safe Labor study conducted between 2002 and 2008, the study investigators noted a Cesarean delivery rate of 11.7% in women with a BMI less than 25 compared with 44.8% in women with a BMI of 40 or greater.[54] In addition, Cesarean delivery is inherently more difficult and complex in obese patients with higher risks of significant intraoperative complications, atony requiring surgical intervention, repeat laparotomy, postoperative infection, venous thromboembolism, and hysterectomy.[53,55]

To date, no randomized controlled trials have been conducted to evaluate the optimal timing of delivery for these patients. Gill and Holbert (2017) used a decision model analysis in a cohort of term obese patients and found that routine induction at 39 weeks was associated with nearly 400 fewer stillbirths, more than 9000 fewer cesarean deliveries, and a cost savings of 30 million dollars compared with expectant management of a hypothetical cohort of 100,000 obese pregnant women.[56] Their decision analysis also suggested a decrease in the number of Cesarean deliveries with routine induction of labor.[56] Lee and colleagues[57] (2016) conducted a retrospective analysis of 74,725 pregnant patients in California and noted that electively induced obese patients were at lower odds of macrosomia, Cesarean delivery, and neonatal adverse outcomes. These findings suggest that induction of labor scheduled for 39 weeks may be optimal to decrease the risk of stillbirth and the morbidity associated with Cesarean deliveries among obese women; however, future research is required before such a recommendation can be made.

With regard to mode of delivery, obese women are more likely to have a "failed" induction of labor compared with normal weight women, with one study noting an almost doubled rate of a failed induction (29% vs 13%).[58] However, it should be noted that obese women may not follow traditional labor curves and may be more subtle in their inflection point from latent to the active phases of labor.[54] In one study, nulliparous women with a BMI of 40 or higher took 1.2 hours longer to reach 10 cm compared with women with a normal BMI.[54] A longer first stage of labor was observed with increasing BMI in both induced and spontaneous labor with unclear pathophysiology regarding the slow progress in the first stage of labor.[54] In contrast, the second stage of labor has been found to be similar among all BMI categories for nulliparous women.[54,59] The evidence suggests that obstetric care providers should exercise patience and allow for adequate time for obese patients to progress through the first stage of labor in order to increase the chance of a vaginal delivery and avoid the complications of a Cesarean delivery in this population.[53]

FETAL CONSIDERATIONS

Several fetal conditions can place the fetus at risk for adverse outcomes (in particular stillbirth), which would necessitate earlier delivery but within the window of the term period. This is predicated on the rationale that the risk of neonatal morbidity associated with an early term birth is no longer outweighed by the benefits of increasing gestational latency in an inhospitable intrauterine environment.

Fetal Growth Restriction

Fetal growth restriction (FGR) is defined by ACOG as fetuses with an estimated fetal weight that is less than the 10th percentile for gestational age. There are multiple causes ranging from maternal to fetal to placental.[60] The optimization of delivery timing for FGR depends on the underlying cause, estimated gestational age, and clinical findings noted on antenatal fetal testing.[60] Current delivery recommendations are based on umbilical artery flow and concurrent conditions, such as amniotic fluid status and maternal comorbidities. Findings of absent end-diastolic flow or reversed end-diastolic flow typically are delivered in the preterm period, thus out of the scope of this current review.[19]

No randomized controlled trials exist regarding the optimal timing of FGR fetuses. Delivery timing is based on the risks of stillbirth and long-term neurologic sequelae.[40,61,62] FGR fetuses with normal Doppler velocimetries and normal amniotic fluid volume are more likely to represent a constitutionally small fetus with lower risk of stillbirth compared with an FGR fetus with abnormal Dopplers.[62] Weekly antenatal testing with biophysical profiles and delivery between 38 and 39 weeks is therefore favored in this population and may be performed closer to 39 weeks to minimize the risk of neonatal complications.[62] The presence of other concurrent medical or obstetric conditions, such as hypertensive diseases of pregnancy, oligohydramnios at term, or a perceived lack of interval growth, may shift the timing of delivery toward the earlier aspect of the term window.[40]

Fetal Anomalies

An estimated 2% to 3% of pregnancies are complicated by major fetal anomalies.[63] These typically carry minimal potential maternal risk, although conditions that predispose to fetal hydrops may lead to maternal Mirror syndrome and consideration of delivery.[63] Most fetal anomalies do not require a preterm or early term delivery. In fact, most would benefit from additional time for growth and maturation in utero, particularly those that will require surgical intervention in the neonatal period.[40] Some fetal anomalies carry an increased risk of stillbirth or fetal growth restriction.[63] In this subset of major anomalies, an indicated early term delivery may be warranted.[63] However, as a whole, the optimal gestational age for delivery cannot be determined due to the heterogeneity of major fetal anomalies. A multidisciplinary approach including maternal fetal medicine specialists, neonatology, and pediatric subspecialists should be undertaken to assist in the timing of delivery and to facilitate postnatal evaluation and treatment.[40,63] With regard to mode of delivery, most of the congenital anomalies do not require Cesarean delivery with few exceptions (eg, giant omphalocele or open neural tube defects), and this should be considered on an individualized basis.[64]

Twin Gestations

Twin gestations regardless of chorionicity and amnion status carry increased maternal and fetal risks.[40] Delivery of twins primarily focuses on minimizing the risk of stillbirth and neonatal morbidity and mortality compared with their singleton counterparts.[65,66] Although twin gestations represent 3% of all births in the United States, they are responsible for a disproportionate number of preterm births and their inherent complications, particularly due to the risks of preterm labor, preeclampsia, and growth restriction.[67] Delivery timing often depends on these complications. In absence of complications, delivery timing is predicated on the balance between the risk of neonatal morbidity and mortality and the risk for stillbirth. Studies from the National

Center for Health Statistics analyzed nearly 300,000 twin gestations, noting that the lowest delivery time frame for perinatal morbidity was around 37 to 39 weeks.[68] This study also calculated gestation-specific prospective risk of fetal and neonatal mortality and noted that the 2 risks were optimized at approximately 39 weeks gestation.[68] Prior studies have noted that in twin gestations in the term period, the most commonly seen complications were respiratory related and the highest risk of neonatal mortality occurred after 39 weeks gestation.[69] Studies have also shown that the risk of stillbirth ranges from 0.2% to 0.4% between 32 and 38 weeks gestation for twin gestations with even higher rates (1.4%) seen beyond 38 weeks, surpassing those of postterm singleton gestations.[70]

For uncomplicated diamniotic dichorionic (DCDA) twin gestations, current ACOG recommendation is delivery between 38 weeks and 0 days to 38 weeks and 6 days.[19] In a study by Soucie and colleagues[71] (2006) it was found that the risk of neonatal respiratory complications requiring ventilatory support decreases after 38 weeks. This study also identified significant risk of neonatal death with DCDA pregnancies extending after 40 weeks.[71] A randomized controlled trial of uncomplicated twin pregnancies (including both monochorionic and dichorionic gestations) comparing delivery at 37 versus 38 weeks noted no difference in composite adverse infant outcomes.[72] Because there is evidence of increasing risk in twin pregnancies extending past 38 to 39 weeks, twin gestations past this time frame should be considered analogous to a postdate singleton gestation.[66,70] Prolongation of pregnancy past this time-frame incurs increasing fetal risk without compensatory neonatal benefit.[66]

Monochorionic diamniotic (MCDA) twin pregnancies are at considerably higher risk of fetal morbidity and mortality due to the pathophysiology of a shared placental unit when compared with DCDA twins. These complications can include unequal placental sharing, selective growth restriction, twin-twin transfusion syndrome, TRAP sequence, and TAPS. Even in absence of these complications, MCDA twin gestations are at increased risk for stillbirth with a rate of 4.3% after 32 weeks.[66,73] These pregnancies thus require close antepartum surveillance, and ACOG provides guidance that uncomplicated MCDA twins should be offered elective delivery between 34 weeks and 37 weeks and 6 days.[19] A model of shared decision-making is recommended.

Mode of delivery is a key issue and controversy in twin deliveries. Most twins are delivered via Cesarean delivery in the United States with reported Cesarean rates as high as 75%.[65,74] Common reasons cited include breech presentation of the first twin or breech presentation of the second twin with concern for complications related to breech extraction.[74] Planned Cesarean delivery for twin gestations was first popularized by the Term Breech Trial and other observational studies that associated planned Cesarean delivery with reduced risk of adverse outcomes in full-term pregnancies with a fetus in breech presentation.[75–79] Barrett and colleagues (2013) conducted a randomized controlled trial in which women with twin pregnancies and vertex presentation of the first twin were randomized to planned Cesarean delivery or planned vaginal delivery. There was no difference noted with regard to neonatal mortality or significant morbidity.[80] Since then, other studies have emerged that have not shown significant differences in reported outcomes between twins who had planned Cesarean versus vaginal delivery.[74,81,82] Given the increased risks of complications and costs associated with Cesarean delivery in light of new evidence regarding the safety and improved outcomes of vaginal delivery for twins, a trial of labor should be pursued for all twin pregnancies with a cephalic-presenting first twin regardless of presentation of the second twin.

Alloimmunization

Hemolytic disease of the fetus and newborn (HDFN), or red cell alloimmunization of pregnancy, is a condition of significant perinatal morbidity and mortality that can be caused by multiple types of maternal antibodies to fetal antigens.[83] The primary concern in these pregnancies is fetal anemia leading to other severe consequences including neonatal thrombocytopenia, neutropenia, and hydrops fetalis.[84,85] HDFN requires heightened surveillance throughout pregnancy with Doppler velocimetry of the middle cerebral artery when critical titers are reached in order to assess for moderate to severe fetal anemia secondary to an immunologic destructive process.[86] In cases where the MCA Doppler velocimetries are greater than or equal to 1.50 multiples of the median adjusted for gestational age, an intrauterine transfusion can be offered to treat the fetal anemia and prevent its sequelae.[87] Because of the decreasing accuracy of MCA Dopplers beyond 37 to 38 weeks, a final transfusion—if required—is generally timed for approximately 35 weeks with delivery recommended between 37 and 38 weeks.[19,40,86] If transfusions are not required during pregnancy, delivery should still be pursued between 37 and 38 weeks. Vaginal delivery should be pursued in the absence of contraindications.[83,86]

OBSTETRIC CONSIDERATIONS
Prior Uterine Surgery

Many pregnancies are complicated by a history of Cesarean delivery, prior uterine surgery, or complications incurred from either (ie, uterine rupture or uterine dehiscence). In 2018, the Centers for Disease Control and Prevention reported a 31.9% Cesarean delivery rate with a range of 22.7% to 37% when stratified by states, stable over the past 5 years.[88] A preponderance of data exists regarding the risks and benefits of trial of labor after cesarean (TOLAC) versus repeat Cesarean delivery. Adverse maternal complications, such as surgical complications, hysterectomy, and transfusion, are less associated with the gestational age than the clinical situation. Uterine rupture, one of the most morbid maternal complications of TOLAC, is more likely to occur in those attempting labor after 40 weeks of pregnancy when compared with the traditional term range, suggesting that delivery before 40 weeks may reduce this risk.[89–91] There is, however, scant literature regarding the optimal timing of delivery within the term period, as in absence of clinical concerns for uterine rupture of labor, delivery in this setting is not pursued before 39 weeks in order to optimize fetal outcomes.[92,93] Similarly, although no randomized controlled trials exist, retrospective data have also suggested that outcomes for repeat higher order Cesarean deliveries are optimized at 39 weeks.[94,95]

A history of vertical hysterotomy, uterine rupture, myomectomy, and dilation and curettage also carry increased risks of uterine rupture. Based on the premise that the myometrium is weakened after prior surgery or uterine rupture, delivery in these cases is recommended before the onset of spontaneous labor, generally at 37 weeks of gestation to balance early term fetal outcomes against the risk of uterine rupture.[19,40]

In cases of prior myomectomy, the risk of uterine rupture depends on several clinical factors, primarily if there was entry into the endometrial cavity.[96] A large myoma burden can also be used to stratify patients into low or high risk of uterine rupture.[19] The available data regarding this topic are limited in that there are few studies that evaluate if location or size of the myomas removed increase the risk of uterine rupture. Currently, ACOG suggests delivery in the early term period ranging from 37 weeks to 37 weeks 6 days due to the risk of uterine rupture.[19]

Even with the aforementioned considerations in timing of delivery, uterine rupture may still occur with a baseline risk of 0.03% to 0.09% in all deliveries. There is a broad range of recurrence risk of uterine rupture in the literature, although no studies include women attempting labor after a history of uterine rupture.[97] Current guidelines from ACOG recommend elective repeat Cesarean delivery scheduled between 36 and 37 weeks 6 days of gestation in order to avoid the onset of spontaneous labor.[98] Zoe and colleagues[99] (2019) analyzed a theoretic cohort of 1000 pregnant patients with a history of uterine rupture to assess the optimal cost/benefit of timing of delivery with the ultimate conclusion of 34 to 35 weeks and 6 days as the optimal time for repeat Cesarean.

Asymptomatic uterine dehiscence, otherwise known as uterine window or Cesarean scar defect, is an obstetric complication that has become more frequently diagnosed due to the widespread use and improved resolution of ultrasound. Although increasing in prevalence, likely due to the increased rate of Cesarean delivery, its clinical course and outcomes are not well described.[100] There is insufficient evidence for delivery timing, other than to suggest that delivery via Cesarean delivery occur before the onset of labor to avoid the risk of uterine rupture.[100] Similar to other conditions that increase the risk of uterine rupture, delivery in the early term period is likely ideal in order to balance the risk of uterine rupture with neonatal morbidities of prematurity.[74,101]

Chronic Abruption

Chronic abruption is described as intermittent or persistent uterine bleeding in the third trimester without any obvious cause and complicates 0.65% to 10% of pregnancies.[40] This chronic disruption of the uteroplacental interface could theoretically progress and could be potentially catastrophic to the fetus and significant maternal blood loss. In the literature there is considerable heterogeneity of the definition and diagnosis of placental abruption and scant evidence of regrading timing of delivery for the chronic subtype.[102] Future study with standardized definitions distinguishing chronic and acute abruptions are needed for evidence-based delivery timing recommendations.

Isolated Oligohydramnios

Defined as an amniotic fluid index less than or equal to 5 cm or largest vertical pocket measuring less than or equal to 2 cm, oligohydramnios is a risk factor for adverse fetal outcome and may indicate the presence of additional maternal, fetal, or obstetric complications.[103–105] Oligohydramnios diagnosed at term in the absence of other medical or fetal factors is typically not associated with adverse fetal outcomes; however, it has been shown to be associated with increased rates of medical intervention.[105] Spong and colleagues[40] (2011) highlighted that the lack of a uniformly used definition of oligohydramnios has led to a lack in consensus of optimal timing of delivery, ultimately suggesting that in uncomplicated isolated oligohydramnios, delivery at 36 to 37 weeks is recommended. Although no randomized controlled trials exist comparing delivery in the early term period with delivery in the full-term period for isolated oligohydramnios, retrospective studies do suggest improved outcomes with delayed delivery.[40] Karahanoglu and colleagues[106] (2016) demonstrated that intervention in the early term period for isolated oligohydramnios was not associated with improved perinatal outcomes compared with expectant management up until 39 weeks. Moreover, early intervention (not specific to oligohydramnios) was associated with higher risks of Cesarean delivery, newborn jaundice, and adverse neonatal outcomes, whereas delivery in the late term period was characterized by higher rates of meconium-stained amniotic fluid and jaundice.[92,106] For these reasons, SMFM currently encourages using a third trimester MVP of <2 cm for the diagnosis of oligohydramnios rather than an AFI <5 cm. Additional work is needed to further ascertain the optimal timing for isolated oligohydramnios.[19,40,92,106]

History of Stillbirth

Stillbirth, defined as fetal deaths at 20 weeks or greater in gestation, has a prevalence of 3 per 1000 births.[107] An increased risk of recurrence has been shown in women with a history of stillbirth, ranging from 3 to nearly 5 times that of the normal population.[108–110] Antepartum surveillance in subsequent pregnancies is generally recommended due to this risk of recurrence.[107] In absence of complications, delivery is recommended at 39 weeks in order to optimize neonatal outcomes, although many women with this history will desire to be delivered in the early term period due to anxiety. ACOG acknowledges this and recommends a model of shared decision-making with appropriate counseling regarding the risks of neonatal morbidity in the early term period.[107]

SUMMARY

Optimizing timing of term deliveries requires careful consideration of numerous factors in order to ensure the best possible maternal and neonatal outcomes. Current recommendations on optimal timing of delivery are based on a mix of evidence ranging from clinical trials to retrospective studies, meta-analysis, systemic reviews, and expert opinions. In uncomplicated deliveries, the results from the ARRIVE trial and its precursors present a strong argument for induction of labor no earlier than 39 weeks. However, there is a multitude of maternal medical, fetal, and obstetric conditions that may necessitate delivery in the early term period. These decisions involve a careful thought process to weigh the risks of neonatal morbidity due to prematurity with the risks of continuing pregnancy in light of these conditions. More definitive data are needed in the form of large prospective observational and randomized controlled trials.

DISCLOSURE

None.

Best Practices

What is the current practice for optimizing term deliveries?

- Early term deliveries are defined as occurring between 37 weeks 0 days and 38 weeks 6 days and full-term deliveries are defined as occurring between 39 weeks and 0 days and 40 weeks and 6 days.
- Delivery of low-risk patients should occur no earlier than 39 weeks 0 days.
- Medical, obstetric, and fetal indications exist that warrant delivery in the early term period. The decision on when to deliver for specific conditions often involves expert opinion and shared decision-making between patient and provider in order to optimize maternal and fetal indications.

What changes in current practice are likely to improve outcomes?

- Institutional review of indications for delivery in the early term period.
- Close antenatal surveillance of high-risk pregnancies to monitor for changes in both maternal or fetal conditions that may prompt delivery or provide reassurance for pregnancy prolongation.
- Shared decision-making with the patient and multidisciplinary care for pregnancies anticipated to deliver in the early term period.

Major Recommendations

- Nonmedically indicated delivery should be recommended to occur no earlier than 39 weeks and 0 days of gestation (level I and II)
- Timing of medically indicated early term deliveries depend on nature of the condition and must be individualized to a patient's unique case. These management decisions should balance the risks of pregnancy prolongation with the neonatal risks of early term delivery (Level I and II)

Summary Statement

- Nonmedically indicated delivery should occur no earlier than 39 weeks and 0 days; however, there are many conditions that necessitate early term delivery to optimize the balance between maternal and fetal risks.

CLINICS CARE POINTS

- For well-controlled chronic hypertension or pregestational diabetes, delivery may be targeted for 39 weeks in absence of other indications.
- Delivery timing for fetal growth restriction should be based on umbilical artery Doppler findings and estimated fetal weight percentile.All twin pregnancies should be delivered prior to 39 weeks.
- Third trimester oligohydramnios should be defined as MVP < 2 cm rather than AFI < 5 cm.
- For women with a history of stillbirth, delivery timing of a subsequent pregnancy should be based on shared-decision making balancing maternal anxiety with risks of neonatal morbidity in the early term period.

REFERENCES

1. Spong CY. Defining "term" pregnancy: recommendations from the defining "term" pregnancy Workgroup. Jama 2013;309(23):2445–6.
2. Fleischman AR, Oinuma M, Clark SL. Rethinking the definition of "term pregnancy". Obstet Gynecol 2010;116(1):136–9.
3. Obstetricians ACo, Gynecologists. ACOG Committee Opinion No 579: definition of term pregnancy. Obstet Gynecol 2013;122(5):1139–40.
4. Tita AT, Landon MB, Spong CY, et al. Timing of elective repeat cesarean delivery at term and neonatal outcomes. N Engl J Med 2009;360(2):111–20.
5. Committee OPQCW. A statewide initiative to reduce inappropriate scheduled births at 360/7–386/7 weeks' gestation. Am J Obstet Gynecol 2010;202(3): 243.e1-8.
6. Oshiro BT, Henry E, Wilson J, et al. Decreasing elective deliveries before 39 weeks of gestation in an integrated health care system. Obstet Gynecol 2009;113(4):804–11.
7. Main EK. New perinatal quality measures from the National quality Forum, the Joint Commission and the Leapfrog group. Curr Opin Obstet Gynecol 2009; 21(6):532–40.
8. Sakala C, Corry MP. Evidence-based maternity care: What it is and what it can achieve. 2008.
9. Clark SL, Frye DR, Meyers JA, et al. Reduction in elective delivery at< 39 weeks of gestation: comparative effectiveness of 3 approaches to change and the impact on neonatal intensive care admission and stillbirth. Am J Obstet Gynecol 2010;203(5):449.e1-6.

10. O'Rourke TP, Girardi GJ, Balaskas TN, et al. Implementation of a system-wide policy for labor induction. MCN Am J Matern Child Nurs 2011;36(5):305–11.
11. Oshiro BT, Kowalewski L, Sappenfield W, et al. A multistate quality improvement program to decrease elective deliveries before 39 weeks of gestation. Obstet Gynecol 2013;121(5):1025–31.
12. Ehrenthal DB, Hoffman MK, Jiang X, et al. Neonatal outcomes after implementation of guidelines limiting elective delivery before 39 weeks of gestation. Obstet Gynecol 2011;118(5):1047–55.
13. Little S, Robinson J, Puopolo K, et al. The effect of obstetric practice change to reduce early term delivery on perinatal outcome. J Perinatology 2014;34(3): 176–80.
14. Obstetricians ACo, Gynecologists. ACOG committee opinion no. 561: nonmedically indicated early-term deliveries. Obstet Gynecol 2013;121(4):911.
15. Kennedy EB, Hacker MR, Miedema D, et al. NICU admissions after a policy to eliminate elective early term deliveries before 39 weeks' gestation. Hosp Pediatr 2018;8(11):686–92.
16. Grobman WA, Rice MM, Reddy UM, et al. Labor induction versus expectant management in low-risk nulliparous women. N Engl J Med 2018;379(6):513–23.
17. Sinkey RG, Blanchard CT, Szychowski JM, et al. Elective induction of labor in the 39th week of gestation compared with expectant management of low-risk multiparous women. Obstet Gynecol 2019;134(2):282–7.
18. Souter V, Painter I, Sitcov K, et al. Maternal and newborn outcomes with elective induction of labor at term. Am J Obstet Gynecol 2019;220(3):273.e1-11.
19. ACOG. "Medically indicated late-preterm and early-term deliveries. ACOG Committee Opinion No. 764." Obstet Gynecol 2019;133:e151–5.
20. Bacak SJ, et al. "Timing of induction of labor." Seminars in Perinatology 2015; 36(6):450–8.
21. Bateman BT, Bansil P, Hernandez-Diaz S, et al. Prevalence, trends, and outcomes of chronic hypertension: a nationwide sample of delivery admissions. Am J Obstet Gynecol 2012;206(2):134.e1-8.
22. Ram M, Berger H, Geary M, et al. Timing of delivery in women with chronic hypertension. Obstet Gynecol 2018;132(3):669–77.
23. Chahine KM, Sibai BM. Chronic hypertension in pregnancy: new concepts for classification and management. Am J perinatology 2019;36(02):161–8.
24. Hutcheon JA, Lisonkova S, Joseph K. Epidemiology of pre-eclampsia and the other hypertensive disorders of pregnancy. Best Pract Res Clin Obstet Gynaecol 2011;25(4):391–403.
25. Abalos E, Cuesta C, Grosso AL, et al. Global and regional estimates of preeclampsia and eclampsia: a systematic review. Eur J Obstet Gynecol Reprod Biol 2013;170(1):1–7.
26. Mol BW, Roberts CT, Thangaratinam S, et al. Pre-eclampsia. Lancet 2016; 387(10022):999–1011.
27. Dahlstrøm BL, Ellström Engh M, Bukholm G, et al. Changes in the prevalence of pre-eclampsia in Akershus County and the rest of Norway during the past 35 years. Acta Obstet Gynecol Scand 2006;85(8):916–21.
28. Wallis AB, Saftlas AF, Hsia J, et al. Secular trends in the rates of preeclampsia, eclampsia, and gestational hypertension, United States, 1987–2004. Am J Hypertens 2008;21(5):521–6.
29. Khan KS, Wojdyla D, Say L, et al. WHO analysis of causes of maternal death: a systematic review. Lancet 2006;367(9516):1066–74.

30. NICE. Hypertension in Pregnancy. The Management of Hypertensive Disorders During Pregnancy. NICE Clinical Guideline 107. 2011.
31. Bernardes TP, Zwertbroek EF, Broekhuijsen K, et al. Delivery or expectant management for prevention of adverse maternal and neonatal outcomes in hypertensive disorders of pregnancy: an individual participant data meta-analysis. Ultrasound Obstet Gynecol 2019;53(4):443–53.
32. Caughey AB, Valent AM. When to deliver women with diabetes in pregnancy? Am J perinatology 2016;33(13):1250–4.
33. Rosenstein MG, Cheng YW, Snowden JM, et al. The risk of stillbirth and infant death stratified by gestational age in women with gestational diabetes. Am J Obstet Gynecol 2012;206(4):309.e1-7.
34. Niu B, Lee VR, Cheng YW, et al. What is the optimal gestational age for women with gestational diabetes type A1 to deliver? Am J Obstet Gynecol 2014;211(4): 418.e1-6.
35. Viteri OA, Dinis J, Roman T, et al. Timing of medically indicated delivery in diabetic pregnancies: a perspective on current evidence-based recommendations. Am J perinatology 2016;33(9):821–5.
36. Kjos SL, Henry OA, Montoro M, et al. Insulin-requiring diabetes in pregnancy: a randomized trial of active induction of labor and expectant management. Am J Obstet Gynecol 1993;169(3):611–5.
37. Lurie S, Insler V, Hagay ZJ. Induction of labor at 38 to 39 weeks of gestation reduces the incidence of shoulder dystocia in gestational diabetic patients class A2. Am J perinatology 1996;13(5):293–6.
38. Berger H, Melamed N. Timing of delivery in women with diabetes in pregnancy. Obstet Med 2014;7(1):8–16.
39. Brown M, Melamed N, Murray-Davis B, et al. Timing of delivery in women with pre-pregnancy diabetes mellitus: a population-based study. BMJ Open Diabetes Res Care 2019;7(1):e000758.
40. Spong CY, Mercer BM, D'Alton M, et al. Timing of indicated late-preterm and early-term birth. Obstet Gynecol 2011;118(2 Pt 1):323.
41. ACOG. ACOG practice bulletin No. 201: pregestational diabetes mellitus. Obstet Gynecol 2018;132(6):e228–48.
42. Abedin P, Weaver J B, Egginton E. Intrahepatic cholestasis of pregnancy: prevalence and ethnic distribution. Ethn Health 1999;4(1–2):35–7.
43. Glantz A, Marschall HU, Mattsson LÅ. Intrahepatic cholestasis of pregnancy: relationships between bile acid levels and fetal complication rates. Hepatology 2004;40(2):467–74.
44. Rioseco AJ, Ivankovic MB, Manzur A, et al. Intrahepatic cholestasis of pregnancy: a retrospective case-control study of perinatal outcome. Am J Obstet Gynecol 1994;170(3):890–5.
45. Lammert F, Marschall H-U, Glantz A, et al. Intrahepatic cholestasis of pregnancy: molecular pathogenesis, diagnosis and management. J Hepatol 2000; 33(6):1012–21.
46. Smith DD, Rood KM. Intrahepatic cholestasis of pregnancy. Clin Obstet Gynecol 2020;63(1):134–51.
47. Lo JO, Shaffer BL, Allen AJ, et al. Intrahepatic cholestasis of pregnancy and timing of delivery. J Matern Fetal Neonatal Med 2015;28(18):2254–8.
48. Puljic A, Kim E, Page J, et al. The risk of infant and fetal death by each additional week of expectant management in intrahepatic cholestasis of pregnancy by gestational age. Am J Obstet Gynecol 2015;212(5):667.e1-5.

49. Ovadia C, Seed PT, Sklavounos A, et al. Association of adverse perinatal outcomes of intrahepatic cholestasis of pregnancy with biochemical markers: results of aggregate and individual patient data meta-analyses. Lancet 2019; 393(10174):899–909.

50. Palmer KR, Xiaohua L, Mol BW. Management of intrahepatic cholestasis in pregnancy. Lancet 2019;393(10174):853–4.

51. SMFM. Intrahepatic cholestasis of pregnancy explained. Published 2011. Accessed2020.

52. Jacob L, Kostev K, Kalder M. Risk of stillbirth in pregnant women with obesity in the United Kingdom. Obes Res Clin Pract 2016;10(5):574–9.

53. Carpenter JR. Intrapartum management of the obese gravida. Clin Obstet Gynecol 2016;59(1):172–9.

54. Kominiarek MA, Vanveldhuisen P, Hibbard J, et al. The maternal body mass index: a strong association with delivery route. Am J Obstet Gynecol 2010;203(3): 264.e1-7.

55. Smid MC, Vladutiu CJ, Dotters-Katz SK, et al. Maternal obesity and major intraoperative complications during cesarean delivery. Am J Obstet Gynecol 2017; 216(6):614.e1-7.

56. Gill L, Holbert M. Computational model for timing of delivery in an obese population. J Matern Fetal Neonatal Med 2018;31(4):469–73.

57. Lee VR, Darney BG, Snowden JM, et al. Term elective induction of labour and perinatal outcomes in obese women: retrospective cohort study. BJOG 2016; 123(2):271–8.

58. Wolfe KB, Rossi RA, Warshak CR. The effect of maternal obesity on the rate of failed induction of labor. Am J Obstet Gynecol 2011;205(2):128 e1-7.

59. Robinson BK, Mapp DC, Bloom SL, et al. Increasing maternal body mass index and characteristics of the second stage of labor. Obstet Gynecol 2011;118(6): 1309.

60. ACOG. ACOG practice bulletin No. 204: fetal growth restriction. Obstet Gynecol 2019;133(2):e97–109.

61. McIntire DD, Bloom SL, Casey BM, et al. Birth weight in relation to morbidity and mortality among newborn infants. N Engl J Med 1999;340(16):1234–8.

62. Galan HL. Timing delivery of the growth-restricted fetus. Seminars in Perinatology 2011;35(5):262–9.

63. Craigo SD. Indicated preterm birth for fetal anomalies. Seminars in Perinatology 2011;35(5):270–6.

64. Peterson AT, Craigo SD. Fetal anomalies. Evid Based Obstet Gynecol 2019;487–94.

65. Lee YM. Delivery of twins. Seminars in Perinatology 2012;36(3):195–200.

66. Newman RB, Unal ER. Multiple gestations: timing of indicated late preterm and early-term births in uncomplicated dichorionic, monochorionic, and monoamniotic twins. Paper presented at: Seminars in perinatology2011.

67. Martin J, Hamilton B, Sutton P, et al. Births: final data for 2008. Natl vital Stat Rep 2010;59(1):1.

68. Kahn B, Lumey L, Zybert PA, et al. Prospective risk of fetal death in singleton, twin, and triplet gestations: implications for practice. Obstet Gynecol 2003; 102(4):685–92.

69. Bilinski RT, Williams SF. Intrapartum management of twin gestations. Obstet Gynecol 2017;37(4):1–5.

70. Sairam S, Costeloe K, Thilaganathan B. Prospective risk of stillbirth in multiple-gestation pregnancies: a population-based analysis. Obstet Gynecol 2002; 100(4):638–41.

71. Soucie JE, Yang Q, Wen SW, et al. Neonatal mortality and morbidity rates in term twins with advancing gestational age. Am J Obstet Gynecol 2006;195(1):172–7.

72. Dodd JM, Crowther CA, Haslam RR, et al. Elective birth at 37 weeks of gestation versus standard care for women with an uncomplicated twin pregnancy at term: the Twins Timing of Birth Randomised Trial. BJOG 2012;119(8):964–73.

73. Barigye O, Pasquini L, Galea P, et al. High risk of unexpected late fetal death in monochorionic twins despite intensive ultrasound surveillance: a cohort study. PLoS Med 2005;2(6):e172.

74. Fox NS, Cohen N, Odom E, et al. Long-term outcomes of twins based on the intended mode of delivery. J Matern Fetal Neonatal Med 2018;31(16):2164–9.

75. Hannah ME, Hannah WJ, Hewson SA, et al. Planned caesarean section versus planned vaginal birth for breech presentation at term: a randomised multicentre trial. Term Breech Trial Collaborative Group. Lancet 2000;356(9239):1375–83.

76. Hogle KL, Kilburn L, Hewson S, et al. Impact of the international term breech trial on clinical practice and concerns: a survey of centre collaborators. J Obstet Gynaecol Can 2003;25(1):14–6.

77. Hoffmann E, Oldenburg A, Rode L, et al. Twin births: cesarean section or vaginal delivery? Acta Obstet Gynecol Scand 2012;91(4):463–9.

78. Smith GC, Shah I, White IR, et al. Mode of delivery and the risk of delivery-related perinatal death among twins at term: a retrospective cohort study of 8073 births. BJOG 2005;112(8):1139–44.

79. Armson BA, O'Connell C, Persad V, et al. Determinants of perinatal mortality and serious neonatal morbidity in the second twin. Obstet Gynecol 2006;108(3 Pt 1): 556–64.

80. Barrett JF, Hannah ME, Hutton EK, et al. A randomized trial of planned cesarean or vaginal delivery for twin pregnancy. N Engl J Med 2013;369(14):1295–305.

81. Sadeh-Mestechkin D, Daykan Y, Bustan M, et al. Trial of vaginal delivery for twins–is it safe? a single center experience. J Matern Fetal Neonatal Med 2018;31(15):1967–71.

82. Schmitz T, Prunet C, Azria E, et al. Association between planned cesarean delivery and neonatal mortality and morbidity in twin pregnancies. Obstet Gynecol 2017;129(6):986–95.

83. Zwiers C, van Kamp IL, Oepkes D. Management of Red Cell Alloimmunization. Fetal Therapy: Scientific Basis and Critical Appraisal of Clinical Benefits. 2019:91.

84. Nicolaides KH, Thilaganathan B, Rodeck CH, et al. Erythroblastosis and reticulocytosis in anemic fetuses. Am J Obstet Gynecol 1988;159(5):1063–5.

85. Koenig JM, Christensen RD. Neutropenia and thrombocytopenia in infants with Rh hemolytic disease. J Pediatr 1989;114(4 Pt 1):625–31.

86. Kumar S, Regan F. Management of pregnancies with RhD alloimmunisation. BMJ 2005;330(7502):1255–8.

87. Moise K. Intrauterine fetal transfusion of red cells. Waltham (MA): UpToDate; 2018. Available at: https://www.uptodate.com/contents/intrauterine-fetal-transfusion-of-red-cells.

88. CDC. Cesarean delivery rate by state. 2019. Available at: https://www.cdc.gov/nchs/pressroom/sosmap/cesarean_births/cesareans.htm. Accessed May 1, 2020.

89. Hammoud A, Hendler I, Gauthier R, et al. The effect of gestational age on trial of labor after cesarean section. J Matern Fetal Neonatal Med 2004;15(3):202–6.

90. Shipp TD, Zelop C, Cohen A, et al. Post–cesarean delivery fever and uterine rupture in a subsequent trial of labor. Obstet Gynecol 2003;101(1):136–9.

91. Guise J-M, Eden K, Emeis C, et al. Vaginal birth after cesarean: new insights. Evid Rep Technol Assess (Summ) 2010;(191):1.

92. Reddy UM, Bettegowda VR, Dias T, et al. Term pregnancy: a period of heterogeneous risk for infant mortality. Obstet Gynecol 2011;117(6):1279.

93. Salmeen K, Cheng Y, Shaffer B, et al. Induction of labor and VBAC success rates: what is the role of gestational age?: 312. Am J Obstet Gynecol 2011;204.

94. Breslin N, Vander Haar E, Friedman AM, et al. Impact of timing of delivery on maternal and neonatal outcomes for women after three previous caesarean deliveries; a secondary analysis of the caesarean section registry. BJOG 2019; 126(8):1008–13.

95. Robinson CJ, Villers MS, Johnson DD, et al. Timing of elective repeat cesarean delivery at term and neonatal outcomes: a cost analysis. Am J Obstet Gynecol 2010;202(6):632.e1-6.

96. Sutton C, Standen P, Acton J, et al. Spontaneous uterine rupture in a preterm pregnancy following myomectomy. Case Rep Obstet Gynecol 2016;2016: 6195621.

97. Frank ZC, Caughey AB. Pregnancy in women with a history of uterine rupture. Obstet Gynecol Surv 2018;73(12):703–8.

98. Bulletins-Obstetrics CoP. Practice bulletin No. 184: vaginal birth after cesarean delivery. Obstet Gynecol 2017;130(5):e217–33.

99. Frank ZC, Lee VR, Hersh AR, et al. Timing of delivery in women with prior uterine rupture: a decision analysis. J Matern Fetal Neonatal Med 2019;1–7. https://doi. org/10.1080/14767058.2019.1602825.

100. Hunter TJ, Maouris P, Dickinson JE. Prenatal detection and conservative management of a partial fundal uterine dehiscence. Fetal Diagn Ther 2009;25(1): 123–6.

101. Fox NS. Pregnancy outcomes in patients with prior uterine rupture or dehiscence: a 5-year update. Obstet Gynecol 2020;135(1):211–2.

102. Downes KL, Grantz KL, Shenassa ED. Maternal, labor, delivery, and perinatal outcomes associated with placental abruption: a systematic review. Am J perinatology 2017;34(10):0935–57.

103. Phelan J, Smith CV, Broussard P, et al. Amniotic fluid volume assessment with the four-quadrant technique at 36-42 weeks' gestation. J Reprod Med 1987; 32(7):540–2.

104. Rutherford SE, Phelan JP, Smith CV, et al. The four-quadrant assessment of amniotic fluid volume: an adjunct to antepartum fetal heart rate testing. Obstet Gynecol 1987;70(3 Pt 1):353–6.

105. Shrem G, Nagawkar SS, Hallak M, et al. Isolated oligohydramnios at term as an indication for labor induction: a systematic review and meta-analysis. Fetal Diagn Ther 2016;40(3):161–73.

106. Karahanoglu E, Akpinar F, Demirdag E, et al. Obstetric outcomes of isolated oligohydramnios during early-term, full-term and late-term periods and determination of optimal timing of delivery. J Obstet Gynaecol Res 2016;42(9):1119–24.

107. Metz TD, Berry RS, Fretts RC, et al. Obstetric care consensus# 10: management of stillbirth:(replaces practice bulletin number 102, march 2009). Am J Obstet Gynecol 2020;222(3):B2–20.

108. Gordon A, Raynes-Greenow C, McGeechan K, et al. Stillbirth risk in a second pregnancy. Obstet Gynecol 2012;119(3):509–17.
109. Robson S, Chan A, Keane RJ, et al. Subsequent birth outcomes after an unexplained stillbirth: preliminary population-based retrospective cohort study. Aust N Z J Obstet Gynaecol 2001;41(1):29–35.
110. Measey MA, Tursan D'espaignet E, Charles A, et al. Unexplained fetal death: are women with a history of fetal loss at higher risk? Aust N Z J Obstet Gynaecol 2009;49(2):151–7.

Hypertensive Disorders of Pregnancy

Whitney A. Booker, MD, MS

KEYWORDS

- Hypertensive disorders of pregnancy • Preeclampsia • Gestational hypertension
- Eclampsia • Maternal morbidity and mortality • Blood pressure

INTRODUCTION

Hypertensive disorders of pregnancy (HDP) describes a group of diagnoses, including preeclampsia and gestational hypertension, in which there is an elevation of blood pressure in response to the physiologic changes of pregnancy. Typically diagnosed by new-onset rise in blood pressures after 20 weeks' gestation, a multitude of maternal organs can be affected, including the kidneys, brain, and liver. Due to the condition's adverse affects on both maternal and fetal health, early and prompt diagnosis are essential on reducing gestational morbidity and mortality.

Incidence

HDP remains a leading cause of maternal and perinatal mortality and morbidity.[1] Although the exact numbers are unknown due to likely underreporting, worldwide HDP is estimated globally to affect 4% to 8% of all pregnancies.[1,2] Specific to the United States, rates of preeclampsia and gestational hypertension have increased significantly, up to 25% and 18%, respectively.[3] Compared with 1980, risk of developing HDP increased more than sixfold after 2000.[4] In addition to rising rates or diagnoses, pregnancy-related mortality has also been on the rise. In a systematic review of maternal deaths, in Latin America and the Caribbean, HDP was the leading cause (more than one-fourth) of maternal mortality, and followed hemorrhage as the second leading cause of death in developed countries.[5]

Much of the increase in rates of HDP has been attributed to a variety of factors including older maternal age at delivery and increases in obesity.[6,7]

Risk Factors

A variety of factors have been thought to attribute to the increasing rate of HDP (**Box 1**). Preeclampsia has commonly been described as a disease of first-time

The author of this article has no commercial or financial conflicts of interests, and no funding sources was utilized in the composition of this article.
Division of Maternal-Fetal Medicine, Department of Obstetrics and Gynecology, College of Physicians and Surgeons, Columbia University Medical Center, 622 West 168th Street, PH-16, New York, NY 10032, USA
E-mail address: wb2322@cumc.columbia.edu

Box 1
Risk factors for Hypertensive disorders of pregnancy

Increased risk
  Previous history of preeclampsia
  Obesity
  Nulliparity
  Advanced maternal age
  Adolescent pregnancy
  Medical comorbidities (ie: chronic hypertension, systemic lupus erythematosus, pregestational diabetes)
  Multifetal gestation

Decreased risk
  Smoking

---

moms. Some studies have demonstrated a 1.5-fold to 2-fold higher incidence in first pregnancies.[8–11] HDP has also been linked to the extremes of maternal age. And although the risk of preeclampsia has been shown to increase across all ages over the past 2 decades, the largest increases has been seen for women older than 35.[12] In addition, overall risk for severe morbidity in the setting of preeclampsia is highest at the extremes of maternal age. Women aged 40 or older have a twofold higher rate of preeclampsia compared with the general population.[13] In addition, HDP has been reported to be higher in adolescent pregnancies, although is unclear if this is related to lack of adequate prenatal care.[14]

Obesity has previously been demonstrated to be one of the strongest risk factors for preeclampsia. Compared with women with a body mass index (BMI) of 21, the risk of preeclampsia doubled at a BMI of 26 (adjusted odds ratio [aOR] 2.1; 95% confidence interval [CI] 1.4–3.4), and nearly tripled at a BMI of 30 (aOR 2.9; 95% CI 1.6–5.3).[15] This rise in preeclampsia parallels the rising rate of obesity in the United States.[6,7] In addition to obesity, other medical conditions may predispose women to HDP. Women with chronic hypertension are at increased risk for developing chronic hypertension.[16] Specifically, the incidence of hypertension is shown to be increased among women with a diastolic blood pressure of at least 100 mg Hg in early pregnancy.[17]

Systemic lupus erythematosus has been shown to be associated with a variety of adverse pregnancy outcomes, including preeclampsia. Most studies demonstrate a worsening prognosis when there is renal involvement[18] Specifically, lupus nephritis has been shown to be predictive of preeclampsia.[19] Overall, the main risk factor is renal involvement and lupus flares during pregnancy. Women with pregestational diabetes have also been shown to be at increased risk for HDP.[20] Risk of preeclampsia increased significantly with worsening underlying disease. In addition, proteinuria in early pregnancy is associated with marked increase in preeclampsia development.[21]

Certain other fetal conditions of pregnancy predispose woman to preeclampsia. Compared with women with singleton gestation, women with twin gestations have been found to have more than double the risk of both gestational hypertension and preeclampsia.[22] And overall, risk for pregnancy-related hypertensive disease has been found to increase progressively with advancing fetal number from singleton to triplet gestation.[23] Risk factors for listed in **Box 1**.

DIAGNOSIS
Classification of Hypertensive Disorders in Pregnancy

The National Institutes of Health and Working Group on Hypertension in Pregnancy has developed a classification of hypertensive disorders in pregnancy that allows for consistent terminology, diagnosis and management (**Fig. 1**). In utilizing both evidence-based medicine and expert consensus, contemporary approaches to hypertension in pregnancy are established.

Preeclampsia and gestational hypertension are pregnancy-specific syndromes related to a reduction in perfusion to specific organs secondary to vasospasm as well as an activation of the coagulation cascade. However, in chronic hypertension there is established elevations in blood pressure that antedate the pregnancy or before 20 weeks' gestation. This distinction has been established, as noted in chronic hypertension, blood pressure elevation is the cardinal pathologic feature of the disease process. However, in HDP an increase in blood pressure is an underlining sign in the context of a complex multiorgan pathophysiologic process.

Chronic hypertension is defined as hypertension that is present before pregnancy or before 20 weeks' gestation. Hypertension is defined as a systolic blood pressure $\geq$140 mm Hg and/or a diastolic $\geq$90 mm Hg. Traditionally, to secure a diagnosis, it is recommended that 2 elevated blood pressures be confirmed, and this be done at least 4 hours apart. Of note, recent recommendations by the American College of Cardiology and the American Heart Association have changed the diagnostic criteria for hypertension in adults.[24] The reason for these changes were made as a response to evidence-based interventions that reflected long-term cardiovascular risk in adults. In this context, obstetrician gynecologists may see patients carrying a diagnosis of chronic hypertension based on nontraditional criteria.

Gestational hypertension is defined as hypertension that is present after 20 weeks' gestation. This diagnosis is given to a patient who was previously normotensive, but has new-onset findings of a systolic blood pressure $\geq$140 mm Hg and/or a diastolic $\geq$90 mm Hg. As in chronic hypertension, this diagnosis is traditionally secured after measurements are taken on 2 occasions at least 4 hours apart. Although in occasions of measured severe hypertension, the diagnosis can be confirmed within a shorter interval to facilitate timely therapy and management.

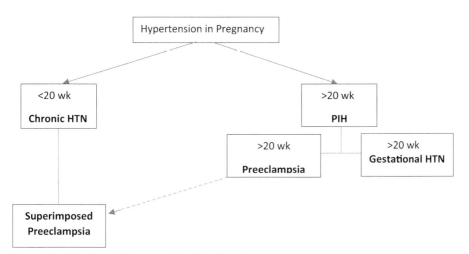

Fig. 1. Classification of hypertensive disorders in pregnancy.

Preeclampsia, like gestational hypertension is defined as hypertension that is, present after 20 weeks' gestation. However in addition to elevations in blood pressure, women with preeclampsia additionally have (1) abnormal laboratory values, (2) symptomatology, or (3) disease-specific physical examination findings. Laboratory values are further discussed later in this article, but may or may not include proteinuria. Symptoms preeclampsia may include headache, blurred vision, scotomata, or abdominal pain. Physical examination findings present may include right upper quadrant pain, abnormal lung sounds consistent with pulmonary edema (rales or crackles), hyperreflexia, and clonus.

Superimposed preeclampsia also described as preeclampsia superimposed on chronic hypertension occurs in women who carry an underlying diagnosis of chronic hypertension and additionally have one of the following:

1. New-onset and/or worsening proteinuria
2. Abnormal preeclampsia syndrome-specific laboratory values
3. Preeclampsia syndrome-specific symptoms
4. Preeclampsia syndrome-specific physical examination findings
5. Sudden increase in blood pressure, which was previously well controlled

Of note, the diagnosis of superimposed preeclampsia may or may not concurrently be associated with severe features. This distinction is important to make, as those women who carry a diagnosis of superimposed preeclampsia can be considered for outpatient management and a later gestational age at delivery.

Severe features of HDP are described in **Box 2**, and can be categorized by (1) blood pressure, (2) symptoms, (3) physical examination findings, (4) laboratory findings.

HELLP Syndrome (hemolysis, elevated liver enzymes, low platelet count) is as severe form of preeclampsia associated with pathologic changes in the liver. These changes include periportal hemorrhages, ischemic lesions, and fibrin deposition. As a result of this liver damage accompanying preeclampsia, there will be abnormalities in serum enzyme levels (aminotransferase and lactate dehydrogenase activities) as well as a low platelet count. In advanced disease processes clinical presentation can also include subcapsular bleeding or even hepatic rupture.[25] Early identification and appropriate management with these patients is essential as maternal morbidity and mortality can be quite high.

Eclampsia is defined as new-onset seizures in the absence of other causative conditions. The seizures can be tonic-clinic, focal, or multifocal. Other causative conditions that must be ruled out include epilepsy, cerebral arterial ischemia and

---

Box 2
Severe features of Hypertensive disorders of pregnancy

	Severe Features
Blood pressure	Systolic blood pressure $\geq$160 mm Hg and/or a diastolic $\geq$110 mm Hg
Symptoms	Headache, blurred vision, scotomata, abdominal pain
Physical examination findings	Right upper quadrant tenderness concerning for HELLP (hemolysis, elevated liver enzymes, low platelet count), abnormal lung sounds consistent with pulmonary edema (rales or crackles), seizure activity
Laboratory values	Transaminitis (aspartate aminotransferase/alanine aminotransferase double the upper limit of normal), thrombocytopenia (platelets <100K), creatinine >1.1

infarction, intracranial hemorrhage, or drug use. In more than two-thirds of cases, eclampsia is preceded by a severe and persistent occipital or frontal headache, blurred vision, photophobia, and altered mental status.[26,27] However, of note, in approximately one-third of cases of eclampsia, women do not demonstrate the classic signs of preeclampsia such as hypertension or proteinuria before the epileptic event.[28]

COMPLICATIONS AND CLINICAL OUTCOMES
Maternal

Women who develop hypertensive disease in pregnancy are at risk for significant maternal morbidity and mortality both antenatally as well as in the postpartum period. Historically, maternal mortality rates in the setting of eclampsia were reported as high as 30%; with the addition of magnesium, antihypertensive medications, and timely delivery, maternal mortality has recently dropped below 1%.[29] But even just having pre-eclampsia with any of the severe features can significantly increase morbidity and mortality.[30] This is important to note because close to 50% of patients presenting with preeclampsia at term progress to preeclampsia with severe features.[31]

In addition to elevations in blood pressure, women often are hypovolemic. This finding of hemoconcentration is important to note, as aggressive attempts to correct with vigorous fluid therapy is often ineffective and can lead to elevations in pulmonary capillary edge pressure and an increased risk of pulmonary edema. Thrombocytopenia is commonly seen[32] and can lead to significant antenatal and postpartum bleeding. Specifically, women with HELLP Syndrome have reportedly significantly higher adverse outcomes in terms of blood products transfusion (25%), disseminated intravascular coagulation (DIC) (15%), wound hematoma (14%), pleural effusion (6%), acute renal failure (35), eclampsia (9%), placental abruption (9%), pulmonary edema (8%), subcapsular liver hematoma (1.5%), and death (1.5%).[33] High rates of blood transfusion are likely due to high rates of placental abruption, DIC, and wound hematomas.

Preeclampsia has been found to be associated with an increased risk of maternal chronic kidney disease, as well as end-stage kidney disease; this risk is significantly higher with preterm preelcampsia.[34] Acutely, women with preeclampsia may have rental deterioration. Due to intrarenal vasospasm, oliguria can occur and result in a 25% reduction in glomerular filtration rate. This commonly occurs in the first 24 hours of the postpartum period.[35]

Hepatic circulation may be decreased due to periportal necrosis. This resultant liver dysfunction can result in a specific risk in aspartate aminotransferase greater than alanine aminotransferase, initially. This may be helpful in differentiating preeclampsia related liver disease from other intrinsic liver pathology (**Table 1**). Liver dysfunction can also results in alterations of normal hepatic synthetic function, resulting in abnormalities in coagulation factors.

Overall, many of the 18 indicators of severe maternal morbidity tracked by the Center for Disease Control and Prevention disproportionally affect pregnancies complicated by preeclampsia; these include stroke, pulmonary edema, heart failure, acute renal failure, and transfusion.[36]

Perinatal

Overall, perinatal mortality rate is higher for infants of women with HDP; and this is regardless of gestational age at delivery.[37] One study demonstrated that in women with HDP, the relative risk for fetal demise was 1.4 compared with normotensive

Table 1
Differential diagnosis for liver diseases in pregnancy

Liver Diseases in Pregnancy	Differentiating Presentations
Hypertensive disorders of pregnancy (including preeclampsia, HELLP [hemolysis, elevated liver enzymes, low platelet count]) Acute fatty liver of pregnancy (AFLP) Viral hepatitis (A, B, C, D, E) Intrahepatic cholestasis of pregnancy Autoimmune hepatitis Primary biliary cirrhosis Gall bladder diseases (biliary colic, acute cholecystitis, common bile duct obstruction, ascending cholangitis, gallstone ileus, pancreatitis)	Pregnancy-specific elevations in blood pressure, elevated aspartate aminotransferase (AST)/alanine aminotransferase (ALT), creatinine, thrombocytopenia, proteinuria Third trimester nausea, malaise, abdominal pain. Elevated AST/ALT, ammonia level and creatinine. Computed tomography (CT) or ultrasound demonstrating fatty liver. Serologic markers for acute and chronic infection Elevated serum bile acids, AST and ALT Often diagnosis of exclusion. Serologic evidence of antinuclear and anti-smooth muscle antibodies is common. Pruritus, elevated serum bile acid levels, alkaline phosphatase. Positive antimitochondrial antibodies; confirmed on liver biopsy Elevated AST/ALT, disease-specific pathology on ultrasound, CT and/or MR cholangiography

Note: This differential is NOT inclusive, but includes several of the more common disease processes seen in pregnancy.

controls. The most common causes of perinatal death were placental abruption and prematurity.[38] Intrauterine growth restriction is also more commonly seen in women with HDP; and this is more common when disease onset is early on and severe.[39]

MANAGEMENT

The cornerstones of managing HDP include prompt diagnosis, antenatal surveillance and treatment, and identifying appropriate timing for delivery

Blood Pressure Management

The goal of therapeutic intervention is to reduce maternal morbidity and mortality; this is specifically to reduce risk of intracranial bleeding and stroke. The ultimate treatment and cure of HDP is delivery of the fetus and placenta. However, initial intervention includes blood pressure management with antihypertensives. Early studies have demonstrated that the risk for intracranial bleeding and stroke are highest for women with a systolic blood pressure greater than 160 mm Hg or a diastolic pressure greater than 105 to 110 mm Hg.[40] In addition, in patients with severe preeclampsia the risk of stroke appears to be higher with severe range systolic hypertension than it is with severe diastolic hypertension.[41] The American College of Obstetricians and Gynecologists (ACOG) recommend that antihypertensive therapy should be initiated expeditiously for acute-onset severe hypertension (systolic blood pressure of 160 mm Hg or more and/or a diastolic blood pressure of 110 mm Hg or more), that is, confirmed as persistent (defined as 15 minutes or more).[35] The goal of treatment is to achieve a blood pressure range of 140 to 150/90 to 100 mm Hg in order to prevent prolonged exposure to severe systolic hypertension, resulting in subsequent loss of cerebral vasculature autoregulation.[42]

The choice of which antihypertensive agent to use requires several considerations. A list of the medications and their doses approved by ACOG are listed in **Table 2**. Intravenous hydralazine or labetalol and oral nifedipine are 3 agents used most commonly in the treatment of acute hypertensive emergencies. Although a Cochrane systematic review found no significant differences regarding either efficacy or safety between hydralazine and labetalol or between hydralazine and calcium channel blockers,[43] other available data suggests that immediate release oral nifedipine maybe considered as first-line therapy.[44–46] This is particularly important when the priority of treatment is expeditious lowering of blood pressure, and IV access may not be readily available. The theoretic concern for concurrent use of nifedipine and magnesium sulfate causing neuromuscular blockage and severe hypotension has been disproven in larger studies.[47] In addition, when IV access has not yet been initiated, a 200-mg dose of labetalol can be administered orally if immediate release oral nifedipine is not available.[48]

In addition to taking into consideration recognized side effects for each of the antihypertensive medications, it is important to note that patients may respond differently to one medication and not another. The non-pregnant medical literature has demonstrated that calcium channel blockers (CCBs) to be more effective in African American patients.[49] Consequently, the National Institute for Health and Clinical Excellence clinical practice guidelines for hypertension recommend CCBs as the initial therapy.[50]

Seizure Prophylaxis

Reduction in seizure risk is best met with timely delivery. However, in addition a large randomized placebo-controlled trial (Magpie study), demonstrated that the rate of seizure was reduced by more than 50% in women who received magnesium sulfate for seizure prophylaxis. Although this is part of the standard prophylactic regimen recommended by ACOG, interestingly, the reduction in seizure activity in those patients receiving magnesium sulfate was not appreciate in women enrolled in high resource settings.[51] In a larger systematic review that followed the Magpie trial, magnesium sulfate not only reduced the rate of seizure activity but also reduced the risk of placental abruption and also maternal mortality as well. They did also notice that the risk of

Table 2 Antihypertensives in pregnancy	
Antihypertensive	**Dose**
Labetalol (IV or oral) Nifedipine (immediate release) Hydralazine	10–20 mg IV, then 20–80 mg every 10–30 min to a maximum cumulative dose of 300 mg *Onset of action 1–2 min* 200 mg po every 12 h, with an increase up to 800 mg every 8–12 h as needed to a maximum cumulative dose of 2400 mg per day *Onset of action 20–120 min* 10–20 mg orally, repeat in 20 min if needed; then 10–20 mg every 2–6 h; maximum cumulative dose of 180 mg *Onset of action within 20 min* 5 mg IV or IM, then 5–10 mg IV every 20–40 min to a maximum cumulative dose of 20 mg *Onset of action 10–20 min*

cesarean delivery was increased by 5% in those patients treated with magnesium sulfate.[52]

In terms of which patients should receive seizure prophylaxis with magnesium sulfate, the evidence is strongest for those with severe features.[53] The 2 randomized trials conducted on those women without severe features reported no cases of eclampsia or progression to severe preeclampsia in those patients who received placebo.[54,55] However, in a larger trial on patients with severe preeclampsia, the rate of seizure activity was 4 times higher in those who did not receive magnesium sulfate.[51]

In some patients (**Box 3**), seizure prophylaxis with magnesium sulfate may be contraindicated or should be used with caution. Other antiepileptics such as benzodiazepines and phenytoin are not as effective in reducing eclamptic seizures[52,56,57] and could only be used in limited circumstances.

Although the eclamptic seizures have occurred at various serum levels of magnesium sulfate, the acceptable therapeutic range recommended by ACOG is 4.8 to 9.6 mg/dL (4–8 mEq/L).[35] The generally accepted regiment in the United States to achieve these levels is administration of an intravenous (IV) bolus of a 4 to 6 g loading dose over 20 to 30 minutes, followed by a maintenance dose of 1 to 2 g/h. Infusion should be continued during the entire intrapartum period (including delivery), and continued postpartum. The ideal duration for continuation during the postpartum period is not clear, but is generally recommended for a period of 12 to 24 hours from delivery. For those patients who are unable to attain intravenous access, magnesium sulfate can be administered intramuscularly with a loading dose of 10 g intramuscular (IM) (5 g IM in each buttock), followed by 5 g every 4 hours. Of note, the incidence of adverse effects has been reported to be higher with intramuscular administration.[51] The commonly experienced adverse effects experienced with magnesium sulfate are often related to serum magnesium levels, and are listed in (**Box 4**). Obtaining serum magnesium levels should be left to the clinical discretion of the provider, but serial examinations assessing the patient's urine output, respiratory status, tendon reflexes are all important indicators of severe toxicity. Decreasing the maintenance dose from 2 to 1 g/h may be indicated in patients with an elevation in creatinine and/or oliguria (less than 30 mL/h over 4 hours).

Antepartum Surveillance

After the diagnosis of HDP (with or without severe features) is confirmed, the decision for antepartum surveillance should be based on gestational age as well as maternal and fetal well-being. Maternal monitoring should include consideration of blood pressure control, onset and duration of clinical symptoms as well as abnormalities in serologic testing. Those patients with severe features should be managed in an inpatient setting, with regular blood pressure monitoring. Patients with severe range blood pressures (systolic $\geq$160 mm Hg and/or diastolic $\geq$110 mm Hg) should be administered antihypertensives. Those patients who are not responsive to antihypertensives

---

Box 3
Contraindications/Cautions in of magnesium sulfate

Myasthenia gravis

Impaired renal function

Myocardial compromise or cardiac conduction defects

Hypocalcemia

Box 4
Side effects of magnesium sulfate

Loss of patellar reflexes

Respiratory depression and paralysis

Cardiac arrest

---

should be precluded from expectant management.[35] Frequency of laboratory testing should be based on the clinical context, but close observation is recommended, as aspartate aminotransferase levels more than 2000 IU/L or lactate dehydrogenase more than 3000 IU/L suggest an increase in mortality risk.[35] Fetal evaluation should include interval ultrasonographic evaluation for fetal weight and amount of amniotic fluid, as well as fetal antepartum testing. Antepartum testing can include a combination of non-stress tests and biophysical profiles; frequency is institutionally dependent.

Indications for Delivery: Maternal Versus Fetal

Indications for delivery are dictated by both risks for the mother versus the fetus in continuing the pregnancy (**Box 5**). In terms of maternal health, the goal is to reduce maternal morbidity and mortality. This includes appropriate antihypertensive management, with the ultimate treatment being delivery of the fetus and placenta. Those patients who are refractory to antihypertensive management, concerning clinical signs and symptoms and/or have laboratory findings concerning for HELLP syndrome are recommended to be delivered regardless of gestational age (see **Box 5**). Two randomized trials demonstrated benefit in those women with HDP with severe features at less than 34 0/7 weeks gestation with reassuring maternal and fetal status to be expectantly managed.[58,59] Expectant management in this cohort of patients has relatively low maternal risk, may prolonged pregnancy by 1 to 2 weeks and can therefore improve neonatal outcomes.[60] Delivery for maternal benefit, may concurrently put the fetus at risk due to associated gestational age-related neonatal morbidity and mortality. In addition, intrauterine signs of fetal compromise including non-reassuring antenatal testing and/or concern for placental abruption indicate that the fetus is at risk; both are contraindications for expectant management.

Box 5
Maternal and fetal indication for delivery in the setting of Hypertensive disorders of pregnancy

Maternal indications for delivery
  Unresponsive to antihypertensives and/or maxed out on 2 antihypertensives
  Clinical signs and symptoms and/or laboratory findings concerning for HELLP (hemolysis, elevated liver enzymes, low platelet count) syndrome
  Persistent headache refractory to treatment
  Visual disturbances and/or altered mental status
  Worsening renal dysfunction
  Pulmonary edema
  Seizure activity

Fetal indications for delivery
  Non-reassuring fetal testing and/or concern for placental abruption
  Intrauterine fetal demise

The decision to deliver is made based on an evaluation of both maternal and fetal risks. Optimal gestational age for delivery depends on the severity of disease process. Expectant management and continued observation is reasonable for those patients with HDP, without severe features.[61] With diagnosis made prior to 37 0/7 weeks, it is reasonable to continue the pregnancy in the absence of abnormal fetal testing, with the of preserving neonatal benefit. This is supported in the largest randomized study, the HYPITAT trial, which assessed women with HDP without severe features after 36 weeks of gestation up until 41 weeks. Women were randomized to expectant management or induction of labor. Those women who were allocated to induction of labor had reduced poor maternal outcomes (new-onset severe preeclampsia, HELLP syndrome, eclampsia, pulmonary edema, placental abruption) compared to those who were allocated to expectant management.[62]

Mode of Delivery

Mode of delivery should be a shared decision-making process between the provider and the patient and should consider multiple factors. In those patients with HDP without severe features, vaginal delivery by induction of labor is preferred. The decision to offer elective cesarean delivery versus trial of labor with induction in patients with severe features who are remote from term should be individualized. Early studies quoted labor induction rates less than 34 weeks as high as 48% when given a chance to delivery vaginally.[63] However, more recent studies in those patients with severe features necessitating delivery between 28 and 32 weeks, likelihood of vaginal delivery is 26.2% and between 24 to 28 weeks 1.8%.[64] Starting Bishop score on admission and advancing gestational age are found to be the best predictors of success.[63] In those patients with hypertension that is, difficult to control and other signs of maternal or fetal compromise, if vaginal delivery is not imminent, cesarean delivery is indicated.

Anesthetic Considerations/Management

Regional anesthesia is the preferred method for women with HDP undergoing labor and delivery. Administration of general anesthesia carries additional risks of aspiration, failed intubation do to pharyngolaryngeal edema and stroke secondary to increased systemic and intracranial pressures during intubation and extubation.[65,66] However, regional anesthesia may be inadequate in the setting of potential hemorrhage and/or coagulopathy where additional anesthetic support may be necessary. Concurrently, thrombocytopenia increases the risk of epidural hematoma. The accepted safe lower-limit for platelet count in the setting of reginal anesthesia is supported only by limited retrospective data, however systematic review from medical literature support the risk of epidural hematoma in a platelet count of 70, 000 to 100,000 is 0.2%.[67] The intrapartum use of magnesium sulfate has been of concern due to its potential to prolong the duration of nondepolarizing muscle relaxants. However, due to the 5-hour half-life of magnesium, discontinuation intrapartum use would only minimally reduced maternal levels while concurrently potentially increasing the risk for eclampsia.[68] Of this reason, magnesium sulfate should be continued during and delivery.

Postpartum Presentations

Gestational hypertension, preeclampsia, and eclampsia can either be persistent from pregnancy or de novo in the postpartum period. Although the incidence of postpartum hypertension is unknown, devastating sequelae-including maternal stroke, seizure, and death[69]-are increasingly common in the postpartum period. Recent studies have demonstrated that in women who sustained hypertensive related stroke, more

Table 3
Clinical risk assessment for preeclampsia

Risk Level	Risk Factors	Recommendation
High	• History of preeclampsia, especially when accompanied by an adverse outcome • Multifetal gestation • Chronic hypertension • Type 1 or 2 diabetes • Renal disease • Autoimmune disease (systemic lupus erythematosus, antiphospholipid syndrome)	Recommend low-dose aspirin if the patient has one or more of these high-risk factors
Moderate	• Nulliparity • Obesity (body mass index >30) • Family history of preeclampsia (mother or sister) • Sociodemographic characteristics (African American race, low socioeconomic status) • Age 35 or older • Personal history factors (eg, low birthweight or small for gestational age, previous adverse pregnancy outcome, more than 10-y pregnancy interval)	Consider low-dose aspirin if the patient has more than one of these moderate-risk factors
Low	• Previous uncomplicated full-term delivery	Do not recommend low-dose aspirin

Reprinted with permission from American College of Obstetricians and Gynecologists. Low-dose aspirin use during pregnancy. ACOG Committee Opinion No. 743. American College of Obstetricians and Gynecologists. Obstet Gynecol 2018;132:e44–52.

than 50% were in the postpartum period.[41] In addition, eclampsia may be most common in the postpartum period, with up to 50% of seizures occurring initially postpartum, most often within 48 hours of delivery.[70,71] Because of this, there is a general consensus that severe postpartum hypertension should be treated.[42] In addition, in women with severe preeclampsia, the administration of postpartum magnesium sulfate to prevent preeclampsia is recommended.[72] The duration of magnesium sulfate and the administration for seizure prophylaxis based on selective criteria of severity to prevent postpartum eclampsia is yet to be determined.[73] In women with HDP, maternal blood pressure has been shown to decrease for the first 2 days postpartum and then increase with a peak from days 3 to 6[74,75]; because of this, it is essential to ensure a women's blood pressure is checked within the first 7 to 10 days postpartum.[76] Severe range blood pressures should be treated, but the preferred antihypertensive medication to be used in the postpartum period is still unclear. The use of nonsteroidal anti-inflammatory medications has recently been brought to concern due to their potential ability to elevate blood pressure. However, data support their safe use in the postpartum patient with blood pressure issues.[77,78]

Management of Future Pregnancies

A variety of preventive strategies have been studied including vitamin supplementation (vitamins C, D, E), fish oil, folic acid, sodium restriction and bedrest; none have demonstrated a significant risk reduction of preeclampsia. In contrast, several clinical trials have demonstrated the beneficial effects of low-dose aspirin. For this reason, ACOG recommends that women with any of the high-risk factors for preeclampsia and those with more than one of the moderate-risk factors should receive a low-dose (81 mg/d) aspirin for preeclampsia prophylaxis initiated between 12 and 28 weeks gestation (**Table 3**).[79] In addition, to date, there are no screening modalities that have been found to play a role in the prediction of HDP.

Long-Term Cardiovascular Risk

Long-term cardiovascular disease (chronic hypertension, myocardial infarction, congestive heart failure), stroke, peripheral artery disease and cardiovascular mortality all remain a significant life time risk for women with a history of HDP.[80,81] The risk of hypertension associated with hypertensive disorders of pregnancy is high immediately after an affected pregnancy and persists for more than 20 years.[82] And women with a history of preeclampsia and eclampsia have approximately double the risk of early cardiac disease and cardiovascular mortality compared to healthy controls.[83] The exact mechanism behind the elevated long-term risk for cardiovascular disease is unclear. Hypertension in pregnancy as well as proteinuria implicate the endothelium as the target of the disease, with subsequent peripheral vasoconstriction and decreased arterial compliance. Endothelial dysfunction, which has also been linked to atherosclerosis, seems to continue in those women with HDP, even after the pregnancy is over.[84] Although elevated lifetime risk factors for hypertension after pregnancy can be explained by prepregnancy risk factors,[85] there seems to also be additionally and endothelial stress antenatally that may play an additional role in increasing a women's risk for cardiovascular disease.[86] For this reason both preventive strategies and close long-term follow-up are key for women with a history of preeclampsia and gestational hypertension.

SUMMARY

In conclusion, HDP remains one of the leading causes of maternal morbidity and mortality worldwide. In most cases, this progression is slow, and the disease can remain slow and without severe features. In other presentations, hypertensive disease and end-organ damage can progress rapidly in just hours. Because of this, prompt diagnosis and close follow-up are essential in the antepartum period. In addition, because of the continued risk in the immediate postpartum period, those at risk should be followed closely. Women with a history of HDP are at increased risk for long-term cardiovascular morbidity and mortality, and so long-term follow-up with a primary care physician is essential.

REFERENCES

1. Steegers EA, von Dadelszen P, Duvekot JJ, et al. Pre-eclampsia. Lancet 2010; 376(9741):631–44.
2. Abalos E, Cuesta C, Grosso AL, et al. Global and regional estimates of pre-eclampsia and eclampsia: a systematic review. Eur J Obstet Gynecol Reprod Biol 2013;170(1):1–7.
3. Wallis AB, Saftlas AF, Hsia J, et al. Secular trends in the rates of preeclampsia, eclampsia, and gestational hypertension, United States, 1987-2004. Am J Hypertens 2008;21(5):521–6.
4. Ananth CV, Keyes KM, Wapner RJ. Pre-eclampsia rates in the United States, 1980-2010: age-period-cohort analysis. BMJ 2013;347:f6564.

5. Khan KS, Wojdyla D, Say L, et al. WHO analysis of causes of maternal death: a systematic review. Lancet 2006;367(9516):1066–74.
6. Flegal KM, Carroll MD, Ogden CL, et al. Prevalence and trends in obesity among US adults, 1999-2008. JAMA 2010;303(3):235–41.
7. Getahun D, Ananth CV, Oyelese Y, et al. Primary preeclampsia in the second pregnancy: effects of changes in prepregnancy body mass index between pregnancies. Obstet Gynecol 2007;110(6):1319–25.
8. Campbell DM, MacGillivray I, Carr-Hill R. Pre-eclampsia in second pregnancy. Br J Obstet Gynaecol 1985;92(2):131–40.
9. Basso O, Christensen K, Olsen J. Higher risk of pre-eclampsia after change of partner. An effect of longer interpregnancy intervals? Epidemiology 2001;12(6): 624–9.
10. Skjaerven R, Wilcox AJ, Lie RT. The interval between pregnancies and the risk of preeclampsia. N Engl J Med 2002;346(1):33–8.
11. Hernandez-Diaz S, Toh S, Cnattingius S. Risk of pre-eclampsia in first and subsequent pregnancies: prospective cohort study. BMJ 2009;338:b2255.
12. Sheen JJ, Huang Y, Andrikopoulou M, et al. Maternal age and preeclampsia outcomes during delivery hospitalizations. Am J Perinatol 2020;37(1):44–52.
13. Duckitt K, Harrington D. Risk factors for pre-eclampsia at antenatal booking: systematic review of controlled studies. BMJ 2005;330(7491):565.
14. Abalos E, Cuesta C, Carroli G, et al. Pre-eclampsia, eclampsia and adverse maternal and perinatal outcomes: a secondary analysis of the world health Organization Multicountry survey on maternal and newborn health. BJOG 2014; 121(Suppl 1):14–24.
15. Bodnar LM, Ness RB, Markovic N, et al. The risk of preeclampsia rises with increasing prepregnancy body mass index. Ann Epidemiol 2005;15(7):475–82.
16. Sibai BM, Lindheimer M, Hauth J, et al. Risk factors for preeclampsia, abruptio placentae, and adverse neonatal outcomes among women with chronic hypertension. National Institute of Child Health and Human Development Network of Maternal-Fetal Medicine Units. N Engl J Med 1998;339(10):667–71.
17. Rey E, Couturier A. The prognosis of pregnancy in women with chronic hypertension. Am J Obstet Gynecol 1994;171(2):410–6.
18. Peart E, Clowse ME. Systemic lupus erythematosus and pregnancy outcomes: an update and review of the literature. Curr Opin Rheumatol 2014;26(2):118–23.
19. Palma Dos Reis CR, Cardoso G, Carvalho C, et al. Prediction of adverse pregnancy outcomes in women with systemic lupus erythematosus. Clin Rev Allergy Immunol 2019. https://doi.org/10.1007/s12016-019-08762-9.
20. Hanson U, Persson B. Outcome of pregnancies complicated by type 1 insulin-dependent diabetes in Sweden: acute pregnancy complications, neonatal mortality and morbidity. Am J Perinatol 1993;10(4):330–3.
21. Sibai BM, Caritis S, Hauth J, et al. Risks of preeclampsia and adverse neonatal outcomes among women with pregestational diabetes mellitus. National Institute of child health and human development network of maternal-fetal medicine units. Am J Obstet Gynecol 2000;182(2):364–9.
22. Sibai BM, Hauth J, Caritis S, et al. Hypertensive disorders in twin versus singleton gestations. National Institute of child health and human development network of maternal-fetal medicine units. Am J Obstet Gynecol 2000;182(4):938–42.
23. Day MC, Barton JR, O'Brien JM, et al. The effect of fetal number on the development of hypertensive conditions of pregnancy. Obstet Gynecol 2005;106(5 Pt 1): 927–31.

24. Whelton PK, Carey RM, Aronow WS, et al. 2017 ACC/AHA/AAPA/ABC/ACPM/ AGS/APhA/ASH/ASPC/NMA/PCNA guideline for the prevention, detection, evaluation, and management of high blood pressure in adults: a report of the American College of Cardiology/American heart association task force on clinical practice guidelines. J Am Coll Cardiol 2018;71(19):e127–248.
25. Weinstein L. Syndrome of hemolysis, elevated liver enzymes, and low platelet count: a severe consequence of hypertension in pregnancy. Am J Obstet Gynecol 1982;142(2):159–67.
26. Sibai BM. Diagnosis, prevention, and management of eclampsia. Obstet Gynecol 2005;105(2):402–10.
27. Cooray SD, Edmonds SM, Tong S, et al. Characterization of symptoms immediately preceding eclampsia. Obstet Gynecol 2011;118(5):995–9.
28. Noraihan MN, Sharda P, Jammal AB. Report of 50 cases of eclampsia. J Obstet Gynaecol Res 2005;31(4):302–9.
29. Sibai BM, McCubbin JH, Anderson GD, et al. Eclampsia. I. Observations from 67 recent cases. Obstet Gynecol 1981;58(5):609–13.
30. von Dadelszen P, Payne B, Li J, et al. Prediction of adverse maternal outcomes in pre-eclampsia: development and validation of the fullPIERS model. Lancet 2011; 377(9761):219–27.
31. Paul TD, Hastie R, Tong S, et al. Prediction of adverse maternal outcomes in pre-eclampsia at term. Pregnancy Hypertens 2019;18:75–81.
32. Giles C, Inglis TC. Thrombocytopenia and macrothrombocytosis in gestational hypertension. Br J Obstet Gynaecol 1981;88(11):1115–9.
33. Audibert F, Friedman SA, Frangieh AY, et al. Clinical utility of strict diagnostic criteria for the HELLP (hemolysis, elevated liver enzymes, and low platelets) syndrome. Am J Obstet Gynecol 1996;175(2):460–4.
34. Barrett PM, McCarthy FP, Kublickiene K, et al. Adverse pregnancy outcomes and long-term maternal kidney disease: a systematic review and meta-analysis. JAMA Netw Open 2020;3(2):e1920964.
35. ACOG practice Bulletin No. 202: gestational hypertension and preeclampsia. Obstet Gynecol 2019;133(1):e1–25.
36. Centers for Disease Control and Prevention. Severe maternal morbidity in the United States. Available at: https://www.cdc.gov/reproductivehealth/ maternalinfanthealth/severematernalmorbidity.html. Accessed March 14, 2020.
37. Plouin PF, Chatellier G, Breart G, et al. Frequency and perinatal consequences of hypertensive disease of pregnancy. Adv Nephrol Necker Hosp 1986;15:57–69.
38. Naeye RL, Friedman EA. Causes of perinatal death associated with gestational hypertension and proteinuria. Am J Obstet Gynecol 1979;133(1):8–10.
39. Odegard RA, Vatten LJ, Nilsen ST, et al. Preeclampsia and fetal growth. Obstet Gynecol 2000;96(6):950–5.
40. Lindenstrom E, Boysen G, Nyboe J. Influence of systolic and diastolic blood pressure on stroke risk: a prospective observational study. Am J Epidemiol 1995; 142(12):1279–90.
41. Martin JN Jr, Thigpen BD, Moore RC, et al. Stroke and severe preeclampsia and eclampsia: a paradigm shift focusing on systolic blood pressure. Obstet Gynecol 2005;105(2):246–54.
42. ACOG committee Opinion No. 767 summary: Emergent therapy for acute-onset, severe hypertension during pregnancy and the postpartum period. Obstet Gynecol 2019;133(2):409–12.
43. Duley L, Meher S, Jones L. Drugs for treatment of very high blood pressure during pregnancy. Cochrane Database Syst Rev 2013;(7):Cd001449.

44. Vermillion ST, Scardo JA, Newman RB, et al. A randomized, double-blind trial of oral nifedipine and intravenous labetalol in hypertensive emergencies of pregnancy. Am J Obstet Gynecol 1999;181(4):858–61.

45. Shekhar S, Sharma C, Thakur S, et al. Oral nifedipine or intravenous labetalol for hypertensive emergency in pregnancy: a randomized controlled trial. Obstet Gynecol 2013;122(5):1057–63.

46. Rezaei Z, Sharbaf FR, Pourmojieb M, et al. Comparison of the efficacy of nifedipine and hydralazine in hypertensive crisis in pregnancy. Acta Med Iran 2011; 49(11):701–6.

47. Magee LA, Miremadi S, Li J, et al. Therapy with both magnesium sulfate and nifedipine does not increase the risk of serious magnesium-related maternal side effects in women with preeclampsia. Am J Obstet Gynecol 2005;193(1): 153–63.

48. Tuffnell DJ, Jankowicz D, Lindow SW, et al. Outcomes of severe pre-eclampsia/ eclampsia in Yorkshire 1999/2003. BJOG 2005;112(7):875–80.

49. Bangalore S, Ogedegbe G, Gyamfi J, et al. Outcomes with angiotensin-converting enzyme inhibitors vs other antihypertensive agents in hypertensive blacks. Am J Med 2015;128(11):1195–203.

50. National Clinical Guideline C. National Institute for Health and Clinical Excellence: guidance. Hypertension: the clinical management of primary hypertension in adults: update of clinical guidelines 18 and 34. London: Royal College of Physicians (UK) National Clinical Guideline Centre.; 2011.

51. Altman D, Carroli G, Duley L, et al. Do women with pre-eclampsia, and their babies, benefit from magnesium sulphate? The Magpie Trial: a randomised placebo-controlled trial. Lancet 2002;359(9321):1877–90.

52. Duley L, Gulmezoglu AM, Henderson-Smart DJ, et al. Magnesium sulphate and other anticonvulsants for women with pre-eclampsia. Cochrane Database Syst Rev 2010;(11):Cd000025.

53. Cahill AG, Macones GA, Odibo AO, et al. Magnesium for seizure prophylaxis in patients with mild preeclampsia. Obstet Gynecol 2007;110(3):601–7.

54. Witlin AG, Friedman SA, Sibai BM. The effect of magnesium sulfate therapy on the duration of labor in women with mild preeclampsia at term: a randomized, double-blind, placebo-controlled trial. Am J Obstet Gynecol 1997;176(3):623–7.

55. Livingston JC, Livingston LW, Ramsey R, et al. Magnesium sulfate in women with mild preeclampsia: a randomized controlled trial. Obstet Gynecol 2003;101(2): 217–20.

56. Duley L, Henderson-Smart DJ, Walker GJ, et al. Magnesium sulphate versus diazepam for eclampsia. Cochrane Database Syst Rev 2010;(12):Cd000127.

57. Belfort MA, Anthony J, Saade GR, et al. A comparison of magnesium sulfate and nimodipine for the prevention of eclampsia. N Engl J Med 2003;348(4):304–11.

58. Sibai BM, Mercer BM, Schiff E, et al. Aggressive versus expectant management of severe preeclampsia at 28 to 32 weeks' gestation: a randomized controlled trial. Am J Obstet Gynecol 1994;171(3):818–22.

59. Odendaal HJ, Pattinson RC, Bam R, et al. Aggressive or expectant management for patients with severe preeclampsia between 28-34 weeks' gestation: a randomized controlled trial. Obstet Gynecol 1990;76(6):1070–5.

60. Magee LA, Yong PJ, Espinosa V, et al. Expectant management of severe preeclampsia remote from term: a structured systematic review. Hypertens Pregnancy 2009;28(3):312–47.

61. Sibai BM. Management of late preterm and early-term pregnancies complicated by mild gestational hypertension/pre-eclampsia. Semin Perinatol 2011;35(5): 292–6.

62. Koopmans CM, Bijlenga D, Groen H, et al. Induction of labour versus expectant monitoring for gestational hypertension or mild pre-eclampsia after 36 weeks' gestation (HYPITAT): a multicentre, open-label randomised controlled trial. Lancet 2009;374(9694):979–88.

63. Nassar AH, Adra AM, Chakhtoura N, et al. Severe preeclampsia remote from term: labor induction or elective cesarean delivery? Am J Obstet Gynecol 1998;179(5):1210–3.

64. Alanis MC, Robinson CJ, Hulsey TC, et al. Early-onset severe preeclampsia: induction of labor vs elective cesarean delivery and neonatal outcomes. Am J Obstet Gynecol 2008;199(3):262.e1-6.

65. Hawkins JL, Koonin LM, Palmer SK, et al. Anesthesia-related deaths during obstetric delivery in the United States, 1979-1990. Anesthesiology 1997;86(2): 277–84.

66. Huang CJ, Fan YC, Tsai PS. Differential impacts of modes of anaesthesia on the risk of stroke among preeclamptic women who undergo Caesarean delivery: a population-based study. Br J Anaesth 2010;105(6):818–26.

67. Lee LO, Bateman BT, Kheterpal S, et al. Risk of epidural hematoma after neuraxial techniques in thrombocytopenic parturients: a report from the multicenter perioperative outcomes group. Anesthesiology 2017;126(6):1053–63.

68. Taber EB, Tan L, Chao CR, et al. Pharmacokinetics of ionized versus total magnesium in subjects with preterm labor and preeclampsia. Am J Obstet Gynecol 2002;186(5):1017–21.

69. Lewis G. Maternal mortality in the developing world: why do mothers really die? Obstet Med 2008;1(1):2–6.

70. Douglas KA, Redman CW. Eclampsia in the United Kingdom. BMJ 1994; 309(6966):1395–400.

71. Matthys LA, Coppage KH, Lambers DS, et al. Delayed postpartum preeclampsia: an experience of 151 cases. Am J Obstet Gynecol 2004;190(5):1464–6.

72. Hypertension in pregnancy. Report of the American College of Obstetricians and Gynecologists' task force on hypertension in pregnancy. Obstet Gynecol 2013; 122(5):1122–31.

73. Vigil-De Gracia P, Ludmir J. The use of magnesium sulfate for women with severe preeclampsia or eclampsia diagnosed during the postpartum period. J Matern Fetal Neonatal Med 2015;28(18):2207–9.

74. Podymow T, August P. Postpartum course of gestational hypertension and preeclampsia. Hypertens Pregnancy 2010;29(3):294–300.

75. Al-Safi Z, Imudia AN, Filetti LC, et al. Delayed postpartum preeclampsia and eclampsia: demographics, clinical course, and complications. Obstet Gynecol 2011;118(5):1102–7.

76. Bernstein PS, Martin JN Jr, Barton JR, et al. National partnership for maternal safety: consensus bundle on severe hypertension during pregnancy and the postpartum period. Obstet Gynecol 2017;130(2):347–57.

77. Blue NR, Murray-Krezan C, Drake-Lavelle S, et al. Effect of ibuprofen vs acetaminophen on postpartum hypertension in preeclampsia with severe features: a double-masked, randomized controlled trial. Am J Obstet Gynecol 2018; 218(6):616.e1-8.

78. Viteri OA, England JA, Alrais MA, et al. Association of nonsteroidal antiinflammatory drugs and postpartum hypertension in women with preeclampsia with severe features. Obstet Gynecol 2017;130(4):830–5.
79. ACOG committee Opinion No. 743: low-dose aspirin use during pregnancy. Obstet Gynecol 2018;132(1):e44–52.
80. Stuart JJ, Tanz LJ, Missmer SA, et al. Hypertensive disorders of pregnancy and maternal cardiovascular disease risk factor development: an observational cohort study. Ann Intern Med 2018;169(4):224–32.
81. Brown MC, Best KE, Pearce MS, et al. Cardiovascular disease risk in women with pre-eclampsia: systematic review and meta-analysis. Eur J Epidemiol 2013; 28(1):1–19.
82. Behrens I, Basit S, Melbye M, et al. Risk of post-pregnancy hypertension in women with a history of hypertensive disorders of pregnancy: nationwide cohort study. BMJ 2017;358:j3078.
83. McDonald SD, Malinowski A, Zhou Q, et al. Cardiovascular sequelae of pre-eclampsia/eclampsia: a systematic review and meta-analyses. Am Heart J 2008;156(5):918–30.
84. Powe CE, Levine RJ, Karumanchi SA. Preeclampsia, a disease of the maternal endothelium: the role of antiangiogenic factors and implications for later cardiovascular disease. Circulation 2011;123(24):2856–69.
85. Romundstad PR, Magnussen EB, Smith GD, et al. Hypertension in pregnancy and later cardiovascular risk: common antecedents? Circulation 2010;122(6): 579–84.
86. Grandi SM, Vallee-Pouliot K, Reynier P, et al. Hypertensive disorders in pregnancy and the risk of subsequent cardiovascular disease. Paediatr Perinat Epidemiol 2017;31(5):412–21.

Contemporary Understanding of Ebola and Zika Virus in Pregnancy

Lauren Sayres, MD[a],*, Brenna L. Hughes, MD, MSc[b]

KEYWORDS

- Emerging infectious diseases • Ebola virus • Zika virus

KEY POINTS

- Pregnancy represents a unique challenge for understanding the emergence of infectious diseases such as Ebola and Zika virus.
- Pregnant women are not at greater risk of acquiring Ebola virus; however, the effects of hypovolemia and hemorrhage are more profound in this population, and pregnancy loss or neonatal demise occurs in nearly 100% of cases.
- Zika virus, typically spread by mosquito vectors, is associated with vertical transmission, resulting in significant congenital defects, namely microcephaly.

INTRODUCTION

The past decade has yielded the emergence of several infectious diseases of critical importance in pregnancy. In particular, the Ebola resurgence of 2013 to 2016 resulted in infection of at least 5000 women of reproductive age and a pregnancy loss rate of nearly 100%.[1] The 2015 to 2016 outbreak of Zika virus captured widespread media attention as 100,000 women of childbearing age became infected, and the significant associated teratogenicity became apparent.[2] Both diseases were determined to be public health emergencies of international concern by the World Health Organization (WHO).[3]

This article seeks to review the epidemiology, transmission, pathogenicity, and management of Ebola and Zika viruses as among the most important emerging infectious diseases in modern history. Our objective is to provide clinically relevant background information and guide best practices for obstetricians as they approach these novel infections.

[a] University of Colorado, Academic Office 1, 12631 East 17th Avenue, Aurora, CO 802, USA;
[b] Duke University Hospital, 203 Baker House, 201 Trent Drive, Durham, NC 27710, USA
* Corresponding author.
E-mail address: laurensayres@gmail.com

Clin Perinatol 47 (2020) 835–846
https://doi.org/10.1016/j.clp.2020.08.005
0095-5108/20/© 2020 Elsevier Inc. All rights reserved.

EBOLA VIRUS
Epidemiology

The genus Ebolavirus is comprised of Ebola virus, Bundibugyo virus, Sudan virus, Taï Forest virus, Bombali virus, and Reston virus.[4] Ebolavirus belongs to the family Filoviridae, which also contains Marburg virus. Ebola virus disease is caused by infection with any of the ebolaviruses, although Bombali and Reston viruses are not known to cause disease in people. Ebola virus was discovered in 1976 in the Democratic Republic of the Congo (formerly Zaire).[5] Ebola virus is associated with an unprecedented high case fatality rate. To date, 17 outbreaks across middle and western Africa have been reported. These outbreaks have led to 15,000 deaths and 34,000 cases, of which at least 5000 cases were among women of childbearing age.[6] The pregnancy-specific mortality rate has been difficult to discern based on published findings but is suspected to be between 74% and 93%.[1,7] The fetal loss rate is nearly 100% for pregnant women with Ebola virus disease.[8,9] Furthermore, of 14 live neonates born to mothers infected with Ebola virus as of 2016, 100% died within 3 weeks of life.[10]

Transmission

The natural reservoir of Ebola virus is unknown, although evidence is accumulating to implicate bats as the most likely source.[11] Most outbreaks in people have been traced back to single spillover events from an infected source. Human-to-human spread of the virus is via direct contact with infected blood and bodily fluids including urine, saliva, stool, vomit, and semen, or from surfaces that have been contaminated with infected fluids.[12] Ebola virus has specifically been identified in amniotic fluid, placental and fetal tissue, and breastmilk.[13-15] Pregnant women are not thought to be at greater risk of acquiring Ebola virus.[16]

Pathogenicity

Ebola virus effectively targets host immune cells, which allows reproduction and dissemination of the virus.[17] The virus inhibits both the innate and adaptive immune responses via inhibition of interferons, impairment of antigen presentation, and neutralization of antibodies against viral glycoproteins. The viral glycoproteins then induce cytopathic effects by damaging endothelial cells and disrupting coagulation pathways, while the activated immune mediators induce cellular apoptosis or necrosis. In particular, these effects result in hepatic, renal, and gastrointestinal injury and coagulopathy. Clinical findings are initially nonspecific and include malaise, myalgia, and fever. As the viral RNA load rises, progression to asthenia, vomiting, secretory diarrhea, and hemorrhage occurs, which without adequate resuscitation can result in hypovolemic shock, multiorgan dysfunction, and death.

There is poor understanding of the specific mechanisms of Ebola pathogenicity in pregnancy. In pregnancy, the effects of hypovolemia and immune dysregulation become exaggerated because of a need for expanded blood volume and an already-altered immune state, respectively.[18] Hypoperfusion of the placenta may represent the mechanism by which miscarriage or intrauterine fetal demise occur. Furthermore, transplacental viral transmission to the amniotic fluid and fetus can result in fetal infection and therefore interruption of normal development and growth.[1,19]

Diagnosis

Diagnosis of Ebola virus can be made presumptively based on symptoms and history of exposure and should be confirmed with molecular testing. Testing typically includes reverse transcriptase polymerase chain reaction (RT PCR) for the detection of viral

RNA in serum, although it is important to note that such tests can be negative for up to 72 hours after symptom onset.[7] Alternatively, enzyme-linked immunoassay (ELISA) testing for immunoglobulin M (IgM) specific to the virus is available, although it is less commonly used, because positive results can be delayed up to 3 weeks in acutely symptomatic patients.[20] Novel rapid diagnostic tests are currently under study but not yet available. Testing strategies remain the same for pregnant women, although rapid testing should be even more imperative given the overlap of the presentation of pregnancy-related conditions and Ebola virus and the potential need for acute obstetric intervention.[7]

Management

The mainstay in management of individuals infected with Ebola virus is supportive management, namely massive fluid resuscitation.[20] Additional measures include frequent monitoring for and correction of electrolyte, glucose, and acid-base imbalances, antiemetic and antidiarrheal therapy, nutritional support, vasopressor support, intubation and ventilation, and continuous renal replacement therapy in the setting of renal dysfunction. Additionally, broad-spectrum antibiotics may be necessary for concomitant infections such as gastroenteritis secondary to bacterial translocation in the setting of gut inflammation or malaria, a frequent coinfection.

There has not been significant research as to the specific care for Ebola virus infections among pregnant women.[21] In 2020, the WHO released guidelines for the management of pregnant women with Ebola virus, which represent the first comprehensive guidelines on specific strategies for their care.[16] When possible, specifically trained providers should be available to care for pregnant women and their neonates, and care should be provided at a private, high-risk facility. Shared decision making for women infected by or recovering from Ebola virus is of necessity.

Generally, maternal rather than fetal indications should take precedent in management decisions. Aggressive fluid resuscitation of up to 10 L per day is particularly important among pregnant women given their significantly increased volume of distribution.[7] There is no strong evidence to suggest that induced abortion, labor induction, or invasive procedures for fetal indications are of benefit to pregnant women with Ebola virus. In fact, fetal monitoring is generally not recommended.[18] There may be benefit to delaying delivery when possible because of the risk of coagulopathy in the setting of high viral load. A decision for surgical delivery should be made on a case-by-case basis, as there is unlikely to be fetal benefit, and women with severe disease may not survive an operation. Fundal massage and administration of uterotonic medications should be strongly prioritized over surgical management of postpartum hemorrhage.[16]

For survivors of Ebola virus who plan pregnancy continuation, comprehensive counseling regarding the risks of fetal or neonatal demise and risk of transmission from pregnancy tissues should be performed.[16] Regular prenatal care with a high-risk obstetrician is recommended for pregnant women who recover from Ebola virus. Expectant management is considered most appropriate.

There is no current approved treatment for Ebola virus. Several therapeutics are undergoing phase I and II clinical trials; these include ZMapp, REGN-EB3, and mAb114 (chimeric monoclonal antibodies) and remdesivir (a broad-spectrum antiviral). Additional antivirals, some of which were designed to target other viruses, are under investigation for use with Ebola virus but have not held as much promise as the aforementioned agents. Convalescent plasma treatment has also demonstrated possible benefit in treatment. The Monitored Emergency Use of Unregistered and Investigational Interventions ethical framework recommends that vulnerable populations including pregnant women be offered similar treatments to the nonpregnant population when potential benefits can outweigh risks. To date, 2 reports describe use of investigational therapeutics in pregnant women with Ebola virus. A 25% mortality rate was noted among 8 women who received convalescent plasma.[22] Additionally, a report details 1 pregnant woman who received favipiravir, a broad-spectrum antiviral, but subsequently died of hemorrhagic shock during labor. However, her newborn is the first reported survivor of congenitally acquired Ebola after receiving ZMapp and remdesivir as well as a buffy coat transfusion from an Ebola virus survivor.[23,24]

Prevention

Critical to the prevention of Ebola virus is interruption of community and healthcare-associated spread.[20] This includes isolation and contact tracing of infected individuals, appropriate containment of infectious material, and protection for those in contact with infected individual.[7] Even if an individual recovers from Ebola virus, a person's bodily fluids may be infectious for 6 months or longer.[25] In particular, pregnancy-related tissue including amniotic fluid, placenta, and fetus are highly infectious even if the pregnant woman has recovered from acute illness. Handling of tissues should be avoided when possible, and potentially infectious waste should undergo proper disposal. Autopsies should be avoided. Personal protective equipment should include a face mask with head cover and eye protection, a gown, double gloves, and boots.[26] Minimization of sharps and invasive procedures can mitigate risk to health care providers.

Multiple trials are underway to study candidate vaccines against Ebola virus.[7] The most promising is the live replicating rVSV-ZEBOV-GP vaccine, which is manufactured by Merck under the trade name Ervebo and has been prequalified by the WHO.[27,28] Although no vaccine, including rVSV-ZEBOV-GP, has been specifically evaluated in pregnant women, an analysis of available data on women who became pregnant during the rVSV-ZEBOV-GP study time frame suggests there to be no significant increase in pregnancy loss or congenital anomalies among vaccinated women.[29] It has been strongly recommended by multiple international public health and humanitarian organizations that pregnant women be included in vaccine clinical trials and compassionate use protocols.[16,30] After years of exclusion from vaccination, pregnant women in the Democratic Republic of the Congo, the location of a widespread Ebola outbreak, were able to start receiving the vaccine in 2019.

ZIKA VIRUS
Epidemiology

Zika virus is a member of the family Flaviviridae, which also includes dengue, West Nile, yellow fever, and Japanese encephalitis viruses.[31] Zika virus was first isolated in 1947 in a Rhesus macaque in the Zika forest of Uganda.[32] Human infection was identified in 1953.[33] There were only 13 cases identified over the next 57 years, until an outbreak affecting 5000 people occurred in Micronesia in 2007.[34] Subsequent outbreaks occurred in Pacific islands, with sporadic cases occurring across Southeast Asia.[35,36] Most recently, a pandemic occurred in Brazil, with virus spreading across the Americas to affect greater than 1 million individuals between 2015 and 2017.[37]

Recognition of the more serious complications of Zika virus began to emerge during the pandemic in Brazil. In particular, approximately 4000 cases of microcephaly were detected in infants of women infected with Zika virus.[38] It has been estimated that 20% to 40% of infected pregnant women will transmit Zika virus to their fetus.[39,40]

Approximately 5% to 10% of cases of vertical transmission will result in fetal loss, and 10% to 15% will result in congenital Zika syndrome including microcephaly. Vertical transmission can occur in any trimester and regardless of maternal symptomatology.

Transmission

Zika virus is spread by multiple species of *Aedes* mosquito to mammalian hosts, including people.[31] The geographic distribution of these mosquito species is expanding secondary to climate change. More recently, it has been discovered that in addition to vectorborne transmission, Zika virus can be spread via sexual contact, perinatal transmission (both during pregnancy and delivery), blood transfusion, and bone marrow and organ transplantation.[41] Although breastmilk has been shown to contain Zika virus, there is no conclusive evidence that the virus can be transmitted by breastfeeding.[42]

Pathogenicity

Zika virus exhibits broad tropism in human cells, undergoing replication and widespread distribution after cell entry by endocytosis.[43] Zika virus preferentially targets neural stem cells and progenitor cells.[44] Zika inhibits the ability of interferons and other cellular signaling pathways to produce an innate immune response to the virus. In pregnancy, Hofbauer macrophages and other immune cells of the placenta that usually serve as a maternal-fetal barrier provide a mechanism for the virus to infect fetal cells.[45]

Zika virus has an incubation period of 3 to 14 days. Most infected individuals are asymptomatic or display mild symptoms such as fever, rash, and myalgias lasting up to 1 week. However, a minority of people will suffer severe neurologic symptoms including meningoencephalitis or Guillain-Barré syndrome because of neurotropism or postinfectious immune response.[46] Given this predilection for neural cells, congenital Zika syndrome is primarily a constellation of central nervous system abnormalities.[47] In particular, fetal brain disruption sequence results in microcephaly and cortical atrophy, intracranial calcifications, other neural and ocular abnormalities, and growth restriction.[48,49] In infants, this manifests with developmental delay, visual or hearing impairment, seizures, and movement and behavioral disorders.[50] It is important to note that asymptomatic pregnant women can still vertically transmit Zika virus to their neonates.

Diagnosis

Zika virus infection is typically detected by serum and urine RT PCR nucleic acid molecular screening and/or serologic IgM ELISA screening.[38] Molecular testing should be performed within 2 weeks of onset of symptoms, whereas serologic testing can be accurately used up to 12 weeks after symptom onset. Of note, serologic testing is subject to significant cross-reactivity with antibodies to other flaviviruses, in particular Dengue virus, and to persistence of antibodies for many months after the resolution of the acute infection.

In nonpregnant individuals with a possible exposure to Zika virus yet without severe symptoms, serum and urine molecular testing are recommended.[51] In the setting of concern for Guillain-Barré, molecular testing of the serum and urine as well the cerebrospinal fluid is recommended as soon as possible. If the index of suspicion for Zika virus infection is high but molecular testing is negative, serum testing for IgM should be performed within 2 to 12 weeks to evaluate for seroconversion.

For pregnant women, the screening paradigm shifts.[52,53] For those with symptoms, serum and urine molecular testing and serologic testing are recommended as soon as possible. If there is a discrepancy with a negative molecular result and positive serologic result, a plaque reduction neutralization serologic test is recommended to confirm infection.[54] Pregnant women with ongoing exposure but no symptoms should be screened with molecular testing every trimester. Dedicated Zika virus testing is not routinely recommended as a routine part of preconception screening or in the setting of a single asymptomatic exposure for pregnant women.

Detailed anatomy ultrasound is recommended at 18 to 22 weeks of gestation for women with symptoms or recurrent exposure, and serial scans should be performed every 3 to 4 weeks thereafter to evaluate for development of evidence of congenital infection.[55] Should there be evidence of fetal anomalies consistent with congenital Zika syndrome on ultrasound, amniotic fluid should be sent for nucleic acid testing if amniocentesis is already being performed for diagnostic purposes. However, amniocentesis is not universally recommended, as a negative result cannot rule out congenital infection caused by the transient and sometimes delayed nature of shedding of the virus into amniotic fluid.[56] If microcephaly or other complex central nervous system abnormalities are noted on routine ultrasound in the absence of alternate explanation and with possible Zika exposure, molecular and serologic testing should be undertaken.

In the setting of suspected congenital Zika infection, newborn or fetus and placenta should be tested after delivery.

Management

Treatment of Zika virus consists of supportive management including antipyretics, analgesics, and rehydration, typically with good response.[38] Severe cases involving Guillain-Barré syndrome may require plasma exchange or immunoglobulin.

There is no approved targeted treatment for Zika virus infection, although several agents are being investigated. These include both host- and virus-targeting antivirals or antibodies, either repurposed from drugs in use for other diseases or screened from compound libraries.[57,58] For example, drugs that upregulate the interferon innate immune pathway or suppress viral replication have shown therapeutic promise.[57] As of yet, no medication has completed phase II clinical trials.[59,60] Additionally, although there is no drug that is proven to mitigate the effects of Zika infection during pregnancy, studies of neutrally active compounds such as NMDA blockers can potentially modulate the fetal neuronal damage that occurs with vertical transmission.[61]

Prevention

Primary prevention strategies against Zika virus include vector control.[62] To prevent mosquito bites, high-risk outdoor areas and in particular bodies of standing water should be avoided. Long sleeves and pants, mosquito repellant, and mosquito netting should be used in endemic regions.[63] Insect repellants, when used per manufacturers' guidelines, are safe for use among pregnant women.[64] Individuals who may have a Zika virus exposure or have a known infection should also undertake measures to avoid mosquito bites and therefore reduce spread. Standard precautions to prevent nosocomial transmission of Zika virus are also important, although as of 2016, no cases of occupational infection have been documented.[65]

Travel guidelines have evolved as the Zika virus epidemic progressed, and additional research is needed to appropriately inform travel restriction policy.[66] General recommendations have been to avoid travel to high-risk regions during pregnancy or while attempting conception.[67,68] Couples residing in affected areas are advised to delay pregnancy.[69] Those with a known exposure or infection should delay attempts at conception for 2 months for female partners and 3 months for male partners.[52] A pregnant woman whose partner has had an exposure or infection with Zika virus should practice abstinence or consistent condom use for the remainder of the pregnancy.

Efforts are underway to develop a vaccine against Zika virus, although none has yet been approved for use. The most promising vaccine candidates have been shown to induce effective antibodies in mice, and phase I and II clinical trials are in process.[70–72] Among the 20 candidates are DNA vaccines, synthetic peptide vaccines, nanoparticles, and live recombinant and purified inactivated viruses.[73]

DISCUSSION

As one faces emerging infectious diseases such as the novel coronavirus first identified in late 2019, the details of the recent Ebola and Zika virus outbreaks can provide a framework for an approach to new diseases.[74] Understanding of the transmission, maternal and fetal effects, and effective treatment, vaccination, and containment methods are imperative to achieving a successful response from the public health and scientific research communities. Specifically addressing emerging infections in pregnancy is important because of the potential differential impact of infections among pregnant women, the possible effects on the fetus, and the unique prophylaxis and treatment strategies necessary for efficacy and acceptability among pregnant women.[75] Attention must be paid to the successes and failures of the response to the Ebola and Zika outbreaks as physicians strive to provide excellent care for pregnant women who are affected by or at risk for emerging infectious diseases.

Best practices

What is current practice?

- Molecular testing is standard of care for both Ebola and Zika viruses.

- Supportive care including rehydration and antipyretics is necessary for individuals infected with Ebola and Zika virus; there are no targeted therapeutics.

- No vaccines are available. Prevention of Ebola virus includes containment of infected substances and personal protection equipment use, and prevention of Zika virus entails protection against mosquito bites, avoidance of high-risk regions, and delay of childbearing.

What changes in current practice are likely to improve outcomes?

- Development of targeted therapeutics and vaccines can decrease the burden of disease and in particular reduce risk for pregnant women and their offspring.

Major recommendations

- Test individuals who have traveled to endemic areas or have been in contact with individuals infected with Ebola or Zika virus who display associated symptoms. There is a role for testing of asymptomatic individuals with recurrent Zika virus exposure also.

- Successful management of Ebola virus includes aggressive rehydration and intensive care. Delivery timing should be based on maternal rather than fetal indications. Properly dispose of all infected substances and use necessary personal protective equipment to prevent nosocomial and community transmission.

- Pregnant women with Zika virus should undergo serial ultrasounds to evaluate for congenital Zika syndrome, although vertical transmission cannot be prevented once a woman has been infected.

- Uninfected women who are pregnant or considering childbearing should avoid travel to Zika virus endemic areas or unprotected intercourse with infected or exposed partners.

Summary statement

Ebola virus is associated with high mortality and a very high pregnancy or neonatal loss rate. Zika virus carries a risk of congenital Zika syndrome. Treatment of both is limited to management of symptoms; therefore prevention of transmission is critical to avoid adverse outcomes.

Data from Refs.[1,2]

REFERENCES

1. Olgun NS. Viral infections in pregnancy: a focus on Ebola virus. Curr Pharm Des 2018;24(9):993–8.
2. Lowe R, Barcellos C, Brasil P, et al. The Zika virus epidemic in Brazil: from discovery to future implications. Int J Environ Res Public Health 2018;15(1):96.
3. McCloskey B, Endericks T. The rise of Zika infection and microcephaly: what can we learn from a public health emergency? Public Health 2017;150:87–92.
4. Kuhn JH, Adachi T, Adhikari NKJ, et al. New filovirus disease classification and nomenclature. Nat Rev Microbiol 2019;17(5):261–3.
5. Bowen ET, Lloyd G, Harris WJ, et al. Viral haemorrhagic fever in southern Sudan and northern Zaire. Preliminary studies on the aetiological agent. Lancet 1977; 1(8011):571–3.
6. Kuhn JH, Amarasinghe G, Perry DL. Fields virology: emerging viruses. 7th edition. Philadelphia: Wolters Kluwer; 2020.
7. Bebell LM, Oduyebo T, Riley LE. Ebola virus disease and pregnancy: a review of the current knowledge of Ebola virus pathogenesis, maternal, and neonatal outcomes. Birth Defects Res 2017;109(5):353–62.
8. Schieffelin JS, Shaffer JG, Goba A, et al. Clinical illness and outcomes in patients with Ebola in Sierra Leone. N Engl J Med 2014;371(22):2092–100.
9. Baggi FM, Taybi A, Kurth A, et al. Management of pregnant women infected with Ebola virus in a treatment centre in Guinea, June 2014. Euro Surveill 2014;19(49): 20983.
10. Nelson JM, Griese SE, Goodman AB, et al. Live neonates born to mothers with Ebola virus disease: a review of the literature. J Perinatol 2016;36(6): 411–4.
11. Kook RA, Bogovocva M, Ansumana R, et al. Searching for the source of Ebola: the elusive factors driving its spillover into humans during the West African outbreak of 2013-2016. Rev Sci Tech 2019;38(1):113–22.
12. Bausch DG, Towner JS, Dowell SF, et al. Assessment of the risk of Ebola virus transmission from bodily fluids and fomites. J Infect Dis 2007;196(Suppl 2): S142–7.
13. Vetter P, Fischer WA 2nd, Schibler M, et al. Ebola virus shedding and transmission: review of current evidence. J Infect Dis 2016;214(suppl 3):S177–84.
14. Caluwaerts S, Fautsch T, Lagrou D, et al. Dilemmas in managing pregnant women with ebola: 2 case reports. Clin Infect Dis 2016;62(7):903–5.
15. Bower H, Grass JE, Veltus E, et al. Delivery of an Ebola virus-positive stillborn infant in a rural community health center, Sierra Leone, 2015. Am J Trop Med Hyg 2016;94(2):417–9.
16. World Health Organization. Guidelines for the management of pregnant and breastfeeding women in the context of Ebola virus disease. Geneva (Switzerland): 2020. Website (accessed 09/22/20): https://apps.who.int/iris/bitstream/handle/10665/330851/9789240001381-eng.pdf?ua=1.

17. Baseler L, Chertow DS, Johnson KM, et al. The pathogenesis of ebola virus disease. Annu Rev Pathol 2017;12:387–418.
18. Black BO, Caluwaerts S, Achar J. Ebola viral disease and pregnancy. Obstet Med 2015;8(3):108–13.
19. Okoror L, Kamara A, Kargbo B, et al. Transplacental transmission: a rare case of Ebola virus transmission. Infect Dis Rep 2018;10(3):7725.
20. Jacob ST, Crozier I, Fischer WA 2nd, et al. Ebola virus disease. Nat Rev Dis Primers 2020;6(1):13.
21. Haddad LB, Jamieson DJ, Rasmussen SA. Pregnant women and the Ebola crisis. N Engl J Med 2018;379(26):2492–3.
22. van Griensven J, Edwards T, de Lamballerie X, et al. Evaluation of convalescent plasma for Ebola virus disease in Guinea. N Engl J Med 2016;374(1):33–42.
23. Dornemann J, Burzio C, Ronsse A, et al. First newborn baby to receive experimental therapies survives ebola virus disease. J Infect Dis 2017;215(2):171–4.
24. Caluwaerts S. Nubia's mother: being pregnant in the time of experimental vaccines and therapeutics for Ebola. Reprod Health 2017;14(Suppl 3):157.
25. Christie A, Davies-Wayne GJ, Cordier-Lassalle T, et al. Possible sexual transmission of Ebola virus - Liberia, 2015. MMWR Morb Mortal Wkly Rep 2015;64(17): 479–81.
26. World Health Organization. Interim guidance: Interim infection prevention and control guidance for care of patients with suspected or confirmed filovirus haemorrhagic fever in health-care settings, with focus on Ebola. Geneva (Switzerland); 2014. Website (accessed 09/22/20): https://apps.who.int/iris/bitstream/handle/10665/130596/1/WHO_HIS_SDS_2014.4_eng.pdf?ua=1&ua=1&ua=1.
27. Samai M, Seward JF, Goldstein ST, et al. The Sierra Leone trial to introduce a vaccine against ebola: an evaluation of rVSVG-ZEBOV-GP vaccine tolerability and safety during the West Africa Ebola Outbreak. J Infect Dis 2018;217(suppl_1): S6–15.
28. Henao-Restrepo AM, Longini IM, Egger M, et al. Efficacy and effectiveness of an rVSV-vectored vaccine expressing Ebola surface glycoprotein: interim results from the Guinea ring vaccination cluster-randomised trial. Lancet 2015; 386(9996):857–66.
29. Legardy-Williams JK, Carter RJ, Goldstein ST, et al. Pregnancy outcomes among women receiving rVSVDelta-ZEBOV-GP ebola vaccine during the Sierra Leone trial to introduce a vaccine against ebola. Emerg Infect Dis 2020;26(3):541–8.
30. Schwartz DA. Maternal and infant death and the rVSV-ZEBOV vaccine through three recent Ebola virus epidemics-West Africa, DRC Équateur and DRC Kivu: 4 Years of excluding pregnant and lactating women and their infants from Immunization. Curr Trop Med Rep 2019;6:213–22.
31. Hamel R, Dejarnac O, Wichit S, et al. Biology of zika virus infection in human skin cells. J Virol 2015;89(17):8880–96.
32. Dick GW, Kitchen SF, Haddow AJ. Zika virus. I. Isolations and serological specificity. Trans R Soc Trop Med Hyg 1952;46(5):509–20.
33. Macnamara FN. Zika virus: a report on three cases of human infection during an epidemic of jaundice in Nigeria. Trans R Soc Trop Med Hyg 1954;48(2):139–45.
34. Petersen LR, Jamieson DJ, Powers AM, et al. Zika virus. N Engl J Med 2016; 374(16):1552–63.
35. Roth A, Mercier A, Lepers C, et al. Concurrent outbreaks of dengue, chikungunya and Zika virus infections - an unprecedented epidemic wave of mosquito-borne viruses in the Pacific 2012-2014. Euro Surveill 2014;19(41):20929.

36. Cao-Lormeau VM, Roche C, Teissier A, et al. Zika virus, French Polynesia, South Pacific, 2013. Emerg Infect Dis 2014;20(6):1085–6.

37. Hennessey M, Fischer M, Staples JE. Zika virus spreads to new areas - region of the Americas, May 2015-January 2016. MMWR Morb Mortal Wkly Rep 2016; 65(3):55–8.

38. Musso D, Ko AI, Baud D. Zika virus infection - after the pandemic. N Engl J Med 2019;381(15):1444–57.

39. Brasil P, Pereira JP Jr, Moreira ME, et al. Zika virus infection in pregnant women in Rio de Janeiro. N Engl J Med 2016;375(24):2321–34.

40. Shapiro-Mendoza CK, Rice ME, Galang RR, et al. Pregnancy outcomes after maternal Zika virus infection during pregnancy - U.S. Territories, January 1, 2016-April 25, 2017. MMWR Morb Mortal Wkly Rep 2017;66(23):615–21.

41. De Carvalho NS, De Carvalho BF, Fugaca CA, et al. Zika virus infection during pregnancy and microcephaly occurrence: a review of literature and Brazilian data. Braz J Infect Dis 2016;20(3):282–9.

42. Colt S, Garcia-Casal MN, Pena-Rosas JP, et al. Transmission of Zika virus through breast milk and other breastfeeding-related bodily-fluids: a systematic review. PLoS Negl Trop Dis 2017;11(4):e0005528.

43. Fernandez-Garcia MD, Mazzon M, Jacobs M, et al. Pathogenesis of flavivirus infections: using and abusing the host cell. Cell Host Microbe 2009;5(4):318–28.

44. Tang H, Hammack C, Ogden SC, et al. Zika virus infects human cortical neural progenitors and attenuates their growth. Cell Stem Cell 2016;18(5):587–90.

45. El Costa H, Gouilly J, Mansuy JM, et al. ZIKA virus reveals broad tissue and cell tropism during the first trimester of pregnancy. Sci Rep 2016;6:35296.

46. Miner JJ, Diamond MS. Zika virus pathogenesis and tissue tropism. Cell Host Microbe 2017;21(2):134–42.

47. Costa F, Sarno M, Khouri R, et al. Emergence of congenital zika syndrome: viewpoint from the front lines. Ann Intern Med 2016;164(10):689–91.

48. Soares de Oliveira-Szejnfeld P, Levine D, Melo AS, et al. Congenital brain abnormalities and zika virus: what the radiologist can expect to see prenatally and postnatally. Radiology 2016;281(1):203–18.

49. Schaub B, Gueneret M, Jolivet E, et al. Ultrasound imaging for identification of cerebral damage in congenital Zika virus syndrome: a case series. Lancet Child Adolesc Health 2017;1(1):45–55.

50. Moore CA, Staples JE, Dobyns WB, et al. Characterizing the pattern of anomalies in congenital zika syndrome for pediatric clinicians. JAMA Pediatr 2017;171(3): 288–95.

51. Oduyebo T, Polen KD, Walke HT, et al. Update: interim guidance for health care providers caring for pregnant women with possible zika virus exposure - United States (including U.S. territories), July 2017. MMWR Morb Mortal Wkly Rep 2017; 66(29):781–93.

52. Management of patients in the context of zika virus: ACOG committee opinion, number 784. Obstet Gynecol 2019;134(3):e64–70.

53. Papageorghiou AT, Thilaganathan B, Bilardo CM, et al. ISUOG Interim Guidance on ultrasound for Zika virus infection in pregnancy: information for healthcare professionals. Ultrasound Obstet Gynecol 2016;47(4):530–2.

54. Sharp TM, Fischer M, Munoz-Jordan JL, et al. Dengue and Zika virus diagnostic testing for patients with a clinically compatible illness and risk for infection with both viruses. MMWR Recomm Rep 2019;68(1):1–10.

55. Carvalho FH, Cordeiro KM, Peixoto AB, et al. Associated ultrasonographic findings in fetuses with microcephaly because of suspected Zika virus (ZIKV) infection during pregnancy. Prenat Diagn 2016;36(9):882–7.
56. Schaub B, Vouga M, Najioullah F, et al. Analysis of blood from Zika virus-infected fetuses: a prospective case series. Lancet Infect Dis 2017;17(5):520–7.
57. Saiz JC, Oya NJ, Blazquez AB, et al. Host-directed antivirals: a realistic alternative to fight zika virus. Viruses 2018;10(9):453.
58. Basak SC, Majumdar S, Nandy A, et al. Computer-assisted and data driven approaches for surveillance, drug discovery, and vaccine design for the Zika virus. Pharmaceuticals (Basel) 2019;12(4):157.
59. Han Y, Mesplede T. Investigational drugs for the treatment of Zika virus infection: a preclinical and clinical update. Expert Opin Investig Drugs 2018;27(12):951–62.
60. Wilder-Smith A, Vannice K, Durbin A, et al. Zika vaccines and therapeutics: landscape analysis and challenges ahead. BMC Med 2018;16(1):84.
61. Schwartz JP, Costa E. Beta Adrenergic receptor-mediated regulation of cyclic nucleotide phosphodiesterase in C6 glioma cells: vinblastine blockade of isoproterenol induction. J Pharmacol Exp Ther 1980;212(3):569–72.
62. Singh RK, Dhama K, Khandia R, et al. Prevention and control strategies to counter zika virus, a special focus on intervention approaches against vector mosquitoes-current updates. Front Microbiol 2018;9:87.
63. LaRocque RL, Ryan ET. Personal actions to minimize mosquito-borne illnesses, including zika virus. Ann Intern Med 2016;165(8):589–90.
64. Diouf K, Nour NM. Mosquito-borne diseases as a global health problem: implications for pregnancy and travel. Obstet Gynecol Surv 2017;72(5):309–18.
65. Olson CK, Iwamoto M, Perkins KM, et al. Preventing transmission of zika virus in labor and delivery settings through implementation of standard precautions - United States, 2016. MMWR Morb Mortal Wkly Rep 2016;65(11):290–2.
66. Errett NA, Sauer LM, Rutkow L. An integrative review of the limited evidence on international travel bans as an emerging infectious disease disaster control measure. J Emerg Manag 2020;18(1):7–14.
67. Petersen E, Wilson ME, Touch S, et al. Rapid spread of zika virus in the Americas– implications for public health preparedness for mass gatherings at the 2016 Brazil Olympic Games. Int J Infect Dis 2016;44:11–5.
68. Prevention CfDCa. Blood & tissue safety: geographic areas at increased risk for Zika virus transmission through blood or tissue donation. 2020. Available at: https://www.cdc.gov/zika/areasatrisk.html. Accessed September 22, 2020.
69. Ndeffo-Mbah ML, Parpia AS, Galvani AP. Mitigating prenatal zika virus infection in the Americas. Ann Intern Med 2016;165(8):551–9.
70. Modjarrad K, Lin L, George SL, et al. Preliminary aggregate safety and immunogenicity results from three trials of a purified inactivated Zika virus vaccine candidate: phase 1, randomised, double-blind, placebo-controlled clinical trials. Lancet 2018;391(10120):563–71.
71. Gaudinski MR, Houser KV, Doria-Rose NA, et al. Safety and pharmacokinetics of broadly neutralising human monoclonal antibody VRC07-523LS in healthy adults: a phase 1 dose-escalation clinical trial. Lancet HIV 2019;6(10):e667–79.
72. Gaudinski MR, Houser KV, Morabito KM, et al. Safety, tolerability, and immunogenicity of two Zika virus DNA vaccine candidates in healthy adults: randomised, open-label, phase 1 clinical trials. Lancet 2018;391(10120):552–62.
73. Poland GA, Ovsyannikova IG, Kennedy RB. Zika vaccine development: current status. Mayo Clin Proc 2019;94(12):2572–86.

74. Schwartz DA, Graham AL. Potential maternal and infant outcomes from (Wuhan) coronavirus 2019-nCoV infecting pregnant women: lessons from SARS, MERS, and other human coronavirus infections. Viruses 2020;12(2).

75. Meaney-Delman D, Jamieson DJ, Rasmussen SA. Addressing the effects of established and emerging infections during pregnancy. Birth Defects Res 2017; 109(5):307–10.

UNITED STATES POSTAL SERVICE ® — Statement of Ownership, Management, and Circulation (All Periodicals Publications Except Requester Publications)

1. Publication Title	2. Publication Number	3. Filing Date
CLINICS IN PERINATOLOGY	001 – 744	9/18/2020

4. Issue Frequency	5. Number of Issues Published Annually	6. Annual Subscription Price
MAR, JUN, SEP, DEC	4	$312.00

7. Complete Mailing Address of Known Office of Publication (Not printer) (Street, city, county, state, and ZIP+4®)

ELSEVIER INC.
230 Park Avenue, Suite 800
New York, NY 10169

Contact Person
Malathi Samayan
Telephone (Include area code)
91-44-4299-4507

8. Complete Mailing Address of Headquarters or General Business Office of Publisher (Not printer)

ELSEVIER INC.
230 Park Avenue, Suite 800
New York, NY 10169

9. Full Names and Complete Mailing Addresses of Publisher, Editor, and Managing Editor (Do not leave blank)

Publisher (Name and complete mailing address)

DOLORES MELONI, ELSEVIER INC.
1600 JOHN F KENNEDY BLVD. SUITE 1800
PHILADELPHIA, PA 19103-2899

Editor (Name and complete mailing address)

KERRY HOLLAND, ELSEVIER INC.
1600 JOHN F KENNEDY BLVD. SUITE 1800
PHILADELPHIA, PA 19103-2899

Managing Editor (Name and complete mailing address)

PATRICK MANLEY, ELSEVIER INC.
1600 JOHN F KENNEDY BLVD. SUITE 1800
PHILADELPHIA, PA 19103-2899

10. Owner (Do not leave blank. If the publication is owned by a corporation, give the name and address of the corporation immediately followed by the names and addresses of all stockholders owning or holding 1 percent or more of the total amount of stock. If not owned by a corporation, give the names and addresses of the individual owners. If owned by a partnership or other unincorporated firm, give its name and address as well as those of each individual owner. If the publication is published by a nonprofit organization, give its name and address.)

Full Name	Complete Mailing Address
WHOLLY OWNED SUBSIDIARY OF REED/ELSEVIER, US HOLDINGS	1600 JOHN F KENNEDY BLVD. SUITE 1800 PHILADELPHIA, PA 19103-2899

11. Known Bondholders, Mortgagees, and Other Security Holders Owning or Holding 1 Percent or More of Total Amount of Bonds, Mortgages, or Other Securities. If none, check box ▶ ☐ None

Full Name	Complete Mailing Address
N/A	

12. Tax Status. (For completion by nonprofit organizations authorized to mail at nonprofit rates) (Check one)
The purpose, function, and nonprofit status of this organization and the exempt status for federal income tax purposes:
☒ Has Not Changed During Preceding 12 Months
☐ Has Changed During Preceding 12 Months (Publisher must submit explanation of change with this statement)

PS Form **3526**, July 2014 [Page 1 of 4 (see instructions page 4)]   PSN: 7530-01-000-9931   PRIVACY NOTICE: See our privacy policy on www.usps.com

---

13. Publication Title		14. Issue Date for Circulation Data Below
CLINICS IN PERINATOLOGY		JUNE 2020

15. Extent and Nature of Circulation		Average No. Copies Each Issue During Preceding 12 Months	No. Copies of Single Issue Published Nearest to Filing Date
a. Total Number of Copies (Net press run)		564	492
b. Paid Circulation (By Mail and Outside the Mail)	(1) Mailed Outside-County Paid Subscriptions Stated on PS Form 3541 (Include paid distribution above nominal rate, advertiser's proof copies, and exchange copies)	427	378
	(2) Mailed In-County Paid Subscriptions Stated on PS Form 3541 (Include paid distribution above nominal rate, advertiser's proof copies, and exchange copies)	0	0
	(3) Paid Distribution Outside the Mails Including Sales Through Dealers and Carriers, Street Vendors, Counter Sales, and Other Paid Distribution Outside USPS®	103	77
	(4) Paid Distribution by Other Classes of Mail Through the USPS (e.g., First-Class Mail®)	0	0
c. Total Paid Distribution (Sum of 15b (1), (2), (3), and (4))	▶	530	455
d. Free or Nominal Rate Distribution (By Mail and Outside the Mail)	(1) Free or Nominal Rate Outside-County Copies included on PS Form 3541	16	19
	(2) Free or Nominal Rate In-County Copies Included on PS Form 3541	0	0
	(3) Free or Nominal Rate Copies Mailed at Other Classes Through the USPS (e.g., First-Class Mail)	0	0
	(4) Free or Nominal Rate Distribution Outside the Mail (Carriers or other means)	0	0
e. Total Free or Nominal Rate Distribution (Sum of 15d (1), (2), (3) and (4))	▶	16	19
f. Total Distribution (Sum of 15c and 15e)	▶	546	474
g. Copies not Distributed (See Instructions to Publishers #4 (page #3))	▶	18	18
h. Total (Sum of 15f and g)	▶	564	492
i. Percent Paid (15c divided by 15f times 100)	▶	97.06%	95.99%

* If you are claiming electronic copies, go to line 16 on page 3. If you are not claiming electronic copies, skip to line 17 on page 3.

UNITED STATES POSTAL SERVICE ® — Statement of Ownership, Management, and Circulation (All Periodicals Publications Except Requester Publications)

16. Electronic Copy Circulation	Average No. Copies Each Issue During Preceding 12 Months	No. Copies of Single Issue Published Nearest to Filing Date
a. Paid Electronic Copies	▶	
b. Total Paid Print Copies (Line 15c) + Paid Electronic Copies (Line 16a)	▶	
c. Total Print Distribution (Line 15f) + Paid Electronic Copies (Line 16a)	▶	
d. Percent Paid (Both Print & Electronic Copies) (16b divided by 16c × 100)	▶	

☒ I certify that 50% of all my distributed copies (electronic and print) are paid above a nominal price.

17. Publication of Statement of Ownership
☒ If the publication is a general publication, publication of this statement is required. Will be printed   ☐ Publication not required.
in the DECEMBER 2020 issue of this publication.

18. Signature and Title of Editor, Publisher, Business Manager, or Owner

Malathi Samayan - Distribution Controller

Malathi Samayan   Date: 9/18/2020

I certify that all information furnished on this form is true and complete. I understand that anyone who furnishes false or misleading information on this form or who omits material or information requested on the form may be subject to criminal sanctions (including fines and imprisonment) and/or civil sanctions (including civil penalties).

PS Form **3526**, July 2014 (Page 2 of 4)   PRIVACY NOTICE: See our privacy policy on www.usps.com

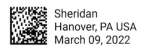